THE HAIR CARE HANDBOOK:

Easy-to-Follow Methods for Beginners to Achieve Healthy Hair, and Easily Mastering Different Styles

Sophia Forbes

CONTENTS

Title Page
Introduction ... 1
Chapter 1: Understanding Your Hair ... 3
Chapter 2: Building a Healthy Hair Care Routine ... 15
Chapter 3: Hair Washing Techniques and Tips ... 25
Chapter 4: Styling Techniques for Beginners ... 35
Chapter 5: Advanced Styling Techniques ... 50
Chapter 6: Protective Styles and Maintenance ... 68
Chapter 7: Addressing Common Hair Problems ... 81
Chapter 8: Natural Hair Care Methods ... 94
Chapter 9: Inspiring Confidence and Creativity ... 107
Conclusion ... 118
References ... 121

INTRODUCTION

Alright, let's get real for a moment. Hair care has always seemed like some mystical quest reserved for those with endless time and secret knowledge. I used to think the same. When I was growing up, my thick hair felt like a curse. Brushing it was a full-on workout. Each tug felt like my scalp was being ripped apart, and let's not even talk about the hair that would come out with each stroke. I'd flip through magazines and read endless online articles to find that magical tip that would change everything. Spoiler alert: it never came.

But here's the good news. Hair care doesn't have to be a labyrinth. This book is here to make it simple, fun, and doable. "The Hair Care Handbook" is designed for teens and young adults who, like me, have struggled to understand all the advice. We will cut through the nonsense and get to what works. We've covered everything from understanding your hair type to mastering styles that make you feel like a rock star.

So, who is this book for? Well, if you've ever felt overwhelmed by your hair, it's for you. It's for you if you've tried a million products and still haven't found "the one." It's for you if you want to rock different hairstyles without spending hours in front of the mirror. If you have hair and want it to look and feel its best, this book is for you.

What makes this book different? For starters, it's written by someone who's been in your shoes. My journey to healthy, manageable hair was a challenging path. It was filled with trial and error. I've researched and tested the methods, and now I'm sharing what works. Plus, we're keeping it real—no jargon, no complicated routines—just straightforward advice you can follow.

Here's what you can expect. The book is divided into easy-to-navigate sections. We'll start with the basics: understanding your hair type and the foundations of good hair care. From there, we'll dive into practical tips for maintaining healthy hair, including choosing the right products and tools. And because we all love a good style switch-up, I'll guide you through various hairstyles, from everyday looks to special occasions. Each chapter has step-by-step instructions, relatable examples, and a dash of humor to keep things light.

This book is about more than just providing you with information. It's about empowering you to take control of your hair health. I want you to feel confident and capable, knowing you have the tools and knowledge to make your hair look amazing. Whether you're dealing with frizz, trying to add volume, or just looking for a fresh style, you'll find the answers here.

And let's remember the fun stuff. Hair care can be a form of self-expression and creativity. It's not just about following rules; it's about experimenting and finding what makes you feel good. This book inspires you to try new things, play with different looks, and enjoy the process.

So, dear reader, let's do this together. Let's transform hair care from a chore into a ritual you look forward to. With the proper techniques, anyone can achieve beautiful, healthy hair. You've got this, and I'm here to help every step of the way.

Welcome to "The Hair Care Handbook." Let's get started on this journey to gorgeous, confident hair!

CHAPTER 1: UNDERSTANDING YOUR HAIR

Have you ever had one of those bad hair days when, no matter what you do, your hair just refuses to cooperate? I remember prepping for a school dance, armed with a curling iron and a dream, only to end up with a frizzy mess that made me look like I'd been electrocuted. Moments like these make you wonder what's going on with your hair. Understanding the science behind your locks can be a game-changer—saving you time, frustration, and a lot of bad hair days. So, let's break it down and get to know what we're dealing with here.

1.1 Hair Anatomy 101: Understanding Hair Structure And Growth

First, let's get a little nerdy and talk about the structure of a hair strand. Picture your hair as a tiny tree. The innermost layer is called the medulla. Not all hair has a medulla, but when it does, it's like the core of an apple—soft and spongy. Its main job is to provide some flexibility. Surrounding the medulla is the cortex, which is the powerhouse of your hair, responsible for its strength and color. Think of it as the sturdy trunk of our tiny tree. The cortex contains the pigment that gives your hair its unique shade, whether blonde, brunette, or rocking a bold color. Finally, the outermost layer is the cuticle. It's a tough, protective shell of overlapping cells, like shingles on a roof. The cuticle's job is to shield the inner layers from damage and keep moisture locked in.

Now, let's talk about hair growth. Have you ever wondered why your hair seems to go through phases where it's growing like a weed and then suddenly stops? That's because hair growth happens in cycles. The first stage is the Anagen phase, the active growth period. Your hair is in "beast mode" during this phase, growing about half an inch per month. Depending on your genetics, this can last anywhere from two to seven years. Next is the Catagen phase, a brief transitional period where growth stops, and the hair follicle shrinks. It's like your hair taking a quick power nap. This phase lasts a few weeks. After that, we enter the Telogen phase, where the hair just chills out. It's a resting phase that lasts around three months, where hair is neither growing nor shedding. Finally, we have the Exogen phase, where the hair sheds to make room for new growth. It's like a seasonal clean-up, making way for fresh, new strands.

There are a few key factors that influence how your hair grows. Genetics plays a huge role in determining the length and thickness of your hair. If your parents have thick, luscious hair, chances are you will be blessed with the same. Hormones also have a significant impact. Puberty, pregnancy, and even menopause can lead to changes in hair growth. You might notice your hair growing faster during pregnancy or shedding more postpartum. Age is another factor. As we age, hair tends to thin out and grow more slowly. It's just a part of the deal.

Maintaining healthy hair follicles is crucial to keep your hair growing strong. This starts with proper scalp hygiene. Think of your scalp as the soil where your tiny trees are planted. Keeping it clean and free from buildup ensures that your hair follicles can do their job effectively. A nutrient-rich diet is also vital. Foods rich in vitamins and minerals, like leafy greens, nuts, and fish, provide the building blocks for healthy hair. And, of course, avoiding harsh chemicals is a must. Opt for gentle, sulfate-free shampoos and conditioners to keep your hair and scalp happy.

Understanding these basics can transform how you approach hair care. It's not just about throwing products at your hair and hoping for the best. It's about knowing what your hair needs and giving it the right environment to thrive. So, buckle up and get ready to become a hair care wizard.

1.2 Identifying Your Hair Type: Straight, Wavy, Curly, And Coily

Alright, let's get into the nitty-gritty of identifying your hair type. Trust me, this is a game-changer. Knowing your hair type can make or break your hair care routine. It's like trying to bake a cake without knowing the ingredients—you'll end up with a mess. So, let's break it down.

First up, we have straight hair, or Type 1. This type of hair lies flat from the roots to the tips, reflecting light to give an enviable shine. Straight hair tends to get oily faster because natural oils from the scalp travel down the hair shaft more easily. Straight hair can range from fine and delicate to thick and coarse but always lacks curl. This type is often the easiest to manage but can be tricky when adding volume or texture. Think of straight hair as a smooth operator of hair types – sleek, shiny, and straightforward.

Next, meet wavy hair, also known as Type 2. Picture gentle, flowing waves that might remind you of beachy curls. Wavy hair strikes a balance between straight and curly. It has a slight bend, forming an S-shape pattern. Type 2A hair is fine and thin with loose, tousled waves. Type 2B hair has more defined waves that start from the mid-lengths, often prone to frizz. Type 2C hair is thick and coarse, with well-defined waves that can start right from the roots. Wavy hair can be a chameleon, offering the versatility of both straight and curly styles. Your waves might behave differently based on the products you use and the weather. Humidity can turn your waves into a frizz fest, but the right products can keep them defined and smooth. It's like having a beach wave look without hitting the surf.

Now, moving on to the curly crowd. Well-defined curls characterize type 3 hair. These curls can range from loose loops to tight ringlets. Type 3A curls are oversized, loose, and often shiny. Type 3B curls are tighter and springier, resembling a corkscrew. Type 3C curls are tight, densely packed, and have a zigzag pattern. Curly hair is bouncy and full of life but can also be high-maintenance. It tends to be drier because natural oils have a more challenging time traveling down the twists and turns of the hair shaft. Curly hair loves moisture, so hydrating products are a must. It's like a sponge—give it enough hydration, and it'll spring to life.

Last but certainly not least, we have coily hair, or Type 4. This hair is the most textured and can be either soft or coarse, forming tight coils or kinks resembling a zigzag pattern. Type 4A hair has dense, springy coils with an S pattern. Type 4B hair has a Z pattern with sharp angles and is prone to shrinkage, meaning it appears shorter than it is because of the tight curls. Type 4C hair has tight coils that are very fragile and need lots of moisture. Coily hair is the most delicate of all hair types and needs extra TLC. Coily hair is incredibly versatile and can be styled in countless ways using protective styles. Still, it thrives on moisture and requires careful handling to avoid breakage. Think of it as a delicate silk fabric that needs careful handling to preserve its complex elegance.

Knowing your hair type is crucial for choosing the right products and styling techniques. Imagine using a heavy, oil-based product on fine, straight hair—a recipe for a greasy disaster. Conversely, using a lightweight product on coily hair might leave it parched and frizzy. Identifying your hair type helps you pick products that complement your hair's natural texture and needs.

So, how do you figure out your hair type? It's simpler than you think. Start with the strand test. Lay a single strand of your hair flat on a white surface. Observe its shape. Is it straight, wavy, curly, or coily? Another method is the texture test. Wash and air-dry your hair without using any products. Once it's dry, examine the texture and pattern. This gives you a clear picture of your natural hair type.

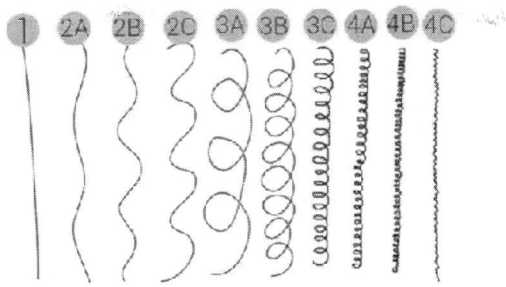

Seeing a visual representation can make it easier to identify your hair. Understanding your hair type opens up a world of possibilities. It's the first step to unlocking your hair's full potential, making your hair care routine more effective and enjoyable. So grab a mirror, do a strand test, and get ready to embrace your hair's natural beauty.

1.3 The Role Of Scalp Health In Hair Care

Let's talk about the unsung hero of hair care—the scalp. Think of your scalp as the foundation of a house. If the foundation is shaky, the whole structure is at risk. A healthy scalp is crucial for hair growth and overall hair health. It's where the magic happens, folks. Nutrients travel through your bloodstream to the hair follicles, delivering the good stuff that keeps your hair growing strong. Scalp circulation is another biggie.

Good blood flow ensures that your hair follicles get all the nutrients they need, kind of like a delivery service for your scalp. But what happens when the scalp is under siege? We've all had those moments where our scalp feels like it's staging a rebellion. Dandruff is a common culprit, making it look like you've been caught in a snowstorm. Those pesky white flakes are dead skin cells shedding faster than usual. Then there's seborrheic dermatitis, which is like dandruff on steroids. It comes with red, itchy patches that make you want to scratch your head. Psoriasis takes it up another notch with thick, scaly patches that can be downright painful. All these conditions can mess with your hair health, making keeping your scalp in tip-top shape crucial.

So, how do you keep your scalp happy? Regular cleansing with gentle shampoos is a must. You don't need anything fancy, just a good, mild shampoo that does the job without stripping your scalp of its natural oils. Scalp massages are another game-changer. They improve blood circulation, helping those nutrients reach where they're most needed. Plus, they feel amazing. Avoid harsh chemical treatments like the plague. They can irritate your scalp and do more harm than good. Stick to products that are kind to your skin.

Scalp treatments can be a lifesaver when things go south. Tea tree oil is an excellent natural remedy for dandruff. It has antimicrobial properties that help keep your scalp clean and flake-free. Aloe vera is fantastic for soothing irritation. It's like a cool drink of water for your scalp, calming things down and reducing redness. Salicylic acid is another goodie. It helps exfoliate dead skin cells, keeping your scalp fresh and healthy. Using these treatments can make a world of difference, transforming a problematic scalp into a healthy one.

Maintaining a healthy scalp isn't rocket science, but it requires some TLC. Think of it as a garden that needs regular watering and care. You can keep your scalp in excellent condition with the proper routine, paving the way for healthy, beautiful hair. Trust me, your scalp will thank you.

1.4 Hair Porosity And Its Impact On Hair Care

Let's chat about hair porosity, the unsung hero of hair care. Imagine your hair as a sponge. How easily it absorbs and retains moisture depends on its porosity. Hair porosity is all about how your hair's cuticle layer—the outermost part—handles moisture. So, why should you care? Because understanding your hair's porosity can be a game changer for your hair routine, making it easier to choose the right products and techniques that work specifically for you.

First up, we have low porosity hair. This type has a tightly packed cuticle layer, which makes it resistant to moisture. Think of it as a sponge that's been dipped in wax. Water and products tend to just sit on top rather than being absorbed. If you've noticed that your hair takes forever to dry or feels greasy even after washing, you might be dealing with low-porosity hair. On the upside, low porosity hair holds on to the moisture it does absorb, but getting it to absorb anything can be a challenge.

Next, let's talk about medium-porosity hair, often referred to as the "Goldilocks" of hair types—everything is just right. The cuticle layer is balanced, allowing moisture to enter and stay, but not too much and not too little. If you have medium-porosity hair, you probably find that your hair dries at a normal rate and responds well to most products. Lucky you! This type is the least fussy and versatile, making it easier to manage and style.

Finally, we have high-porosity hair. This type has gaps and holes in the cuticle layer, making it like a sponge full of holes. It absorbs moisture quickly but loses it just as fast. High-porosity hair can be a result of damage from heat styling, chemical treatments, or genetics. If your hair tends to feel dry, frizzy, and tangled, you might have high-porosity hair. It drinks up the moisture but struggles to retain it, requiring more frequent conditioning and moisturizing.

So, how do you figure out your hair's porosity? It's easier than you think. First, try the float test. Drop a clean strand of your hair into a glass of water. If it floats, you have low-porosity hair. If it sinks slowly, you have medium porosity hair. If it sinks quickly, you have high porosity hair. Another method is the slip test. Run your fingers down a strand of hair. If it feels smooth, you have low-porosity hair. If it feels slightly bumpy, you have medium porosity. If it feels very rough and uneven, you're likely dealing with high-porosity hair.

Knowing your hair porosity has significant implications for your hair care routine. Low-porosity hair needs lightweight products that won't sit on top and cause buildup. Look for water-based products and avoid heavy oils and butters. Medium-porosity hair can handle various products, so you are welcome to experiment and see what works best for you. High-porosity hair needs heavy-duty moisture. Deep conditioning treatments are your best friend, and you should look for products with ingredients like shea butter and oils that can help seal the cuticle.

Understanding your hair's porosity can make your hair care routine a whole lot easier. It's like having a personalized guide to what your hair needs. So, grab that glass of water, do the float test, and get ready to give your hair the love it deserves.

1.5 Understanding Hair Density And Thickness

Alright, let's get into the nitty-gritty of hair density and thickness. These terms might sound interchangeable, but they're quite different. Understanding both can make a huge difference in how you care for and style your hair. Hair density refers to the number of hair strands per square inch on your scalp. Think of it like a crowded subway car—more people (or hair strands) mean higher density. If you've ever looked in the mirror and thought, "Why can I see so much of my scalp?" you might have low-density hair. On the flip side, you likely have high-density hair if your hair feels like a thick forest.

Hair thickness, on the other hand, is all about the diameter of the individual hair strands. Hold a single strand of hair between your fingers. If it feels thin like silk, you have fine hair. If it feels more substantial, you might have medium or thick hair. It's essential to understand both these aspects because they affect everything from how your hair holds a style to how much product you need. For example, thick hair strands might need heavier products to stay moisturized, while fine hair can get weighed down easily.

So, how do you figure out your hair density? A straightforward method is the scalp visibility test. Stand in front of a mirror and look at your scalp. If you can see a lot of it, you have low-density hair. If you can barely see any scalp, you've got high-density hair. Another method is to take a small section of your hair and count the strands. This might sound tedious, but it gives you a clear idea. Grab a one-inch section of your hair and start counting. If you get a high number, you have high-density hair; if the count is low, you know the drill.

Now, let's talk about what affects hair density and thickness. Genetics plays a huge role. If your family tree is full of people with thick, lush hair, chances are you'll have the same. Health conditions like alopecia can also impact hair density, leading to thinning and hair loss. Nutrient deficiencies can mess with your hair's thickness, too. If your diet lacks essential vitamins and minerals, your hair might become finer and less dense. Ensuring you get enough iron, zinc, and vitamins can help keep your hair looking its best.

You've figured out your hair density and thickness—now what? It's time to tailor your hair care routine. If you have low-density hair, volumizing products are your best friends. Look for shampoos and conditioners that add body and lift. When it comes to styling, go for techniques that create the illusion of more volume, like backcombing or using a root-lifting spray. For those with high-density hair, lightweight products are essential. Heavy creams and oils can weigh your hair, making it look flat. Opt for light, hydrating products that won't add extra weight.

For thick hair strands, you'll need products that can penetrate deeply and provide moisture. Thick hair can handle heavier products like butters and oils, which help keep it hydrated and manageable. Fine hair, however, needs a delicate touch. Lightweight sprays and mousses can add volume without making your hair feel greasy. When styling fine hair, avoid heavy products that can cause buildup and make your hair look limp.

Understanding these aspects of your hair can make all the difference. It's like having a custom-made roadmap for your hair care routine. You'll know exactly what your hair needs and how to give it the care it deserves. Armed with this knowledge, you're well on your way to achieving the hair of your dreams.

1.6 Common Hair Myths Debunked

Ah, hair myths. We've all heard them, and some of us have even tried them out, only to be left scratching our heads—literally and figuratively. Let's start with one of the most persistent myths: "Cutting your hair makes it grow faster." I mean, if that were true, wouldn't we all have Rapunzel-length locks by now? The reality is that cutting your hair does not affect its growth rate. Hair growth is determined by genetics, hormones, and overall health, not by how often you trim it. Trimming your hair can make it look healthier by removing split ends, but it won't turn you into a hair-growing machine overnight.

Next, let's tackle the old wives' tale that brushing your hair 100 times daily will make it shiny and healthy. While sitting in front of a mirror, brushing your hair until it gleams might seem soothing, but it's counterproductive. Over-brushing can lead to breakage, split ends, and even hair loss, especially if you are using a typical plastic bristle brush. Instead, opt for a brush with a broad, dense pad of soft-to-medium bristles, which is gentler on your hair. Think of it as polishing a delicate vase—using the wrong tool does more harm than good. Focus on gentle detangling and choose a brush for your hair type. Your hair will thank you for it.

Another myth worth debunking is that shampooing every day is necessary. While some people with oily scalps might benefit from daily washing, most don't need to lather up that often. Over washing can strip your hair of natural oils, leading to dryness and irritation. Instead, find a washing schedule that suits your hair type and lifestyle. Some people do well with washing every other day, while others might find that once or twice a week is sufficient.

Let's discuss the myth that natural hair care products are always better. While it's true that many natural ingredients can benefit your hair, not all natural products are created equal. Some lack the preservatives needed to keep them safe and effective. On the flip side, not all synthetic ingredients are harmful. Many are formulated to be hypoallergenic and effective. The key is to read labels, understand what you're putting on your hair, and choose products that meet your specific needs.

Finally, there's the belief that you should only use one brand of hair care products. This myth likely started as a marketing tactic, but the truth is that mixing and matching can be beneficial. Your hair's needs can change due to weather, diet, and hormonal shifts. You are welcome to experiment with different brands and products to find what works best.

So, where did these myths come from? Many have roots in historical practices and media influence. Back then, people believed frequent haircuts stimulated the scalp and promoted growth. Generations of well-meaning parents and hairdressers have perpetuated this myth. The 100-strokes myth began as a way to encourage good grooming habits in a time when people used pomatums, powders, and oils instead of soap, along with very different brushes. As we transitioned to using soap and shampoo and changed the types of brushes we used, these practices began to cause the problems we see today. Media also plays a significant role, often showcasing glossy, perfectly brushed hair in movies and advertisements, leading us to believe that more brushing equals healthier hair mistakenly.

It's essential to question the advice you hear and seek information from reliable sources. Consult dermatologists and trichologists if you need clarification on a hair practice. Reading scientific studies and articles can also help you separate fact from fiction. For instance, the National Center for Biotechnology Information (NCBI) provides peer-reviewed research on hair growth and health. Staying informed will help you make better decisions for your hair.

Questioning hair care advice and seeking reliable information can make a difference. Don't just take my word for it—do your homework, ask the experts, and remember that your hair is as unique as you are. With some critical thinking and the proper knowledge, you can debunk these myths and take better care of your hair. So go ahead, challenge that age-old wisdom, and embrace a more informed approach to hair care. Your locks will thank you for it

CHAPTER 2: BUILDING A HEALTHY HAIR CARE ROUTINE

Imagine waking up every day with hair that looks like it just stepped out of a shampoo commercial. Sounds like a dream, right? Well, it's not as far-fetched as you might think. Building a healthy hair care routine is like brushing your teeth—small, consistent actions can make a massive difference over time. You don't need to spend hours in front of the mirror or empty your wallet on fancy products. It's all about finding what works for you and sticking to it. Let's dive into the daily essentials that will have your hair looking and feeling its best.

2.1 Daily Hair Care: Essential Steps For Every Day

Maintaining your hair daily is the foundation of healthy locks. It's like watering a plant; a little care every day goes a long way. One of the easiest and most effective things you can do is give yourself a daily scalp massage. Not only does it feel fantastic, but it also boosts blood circulation to your hair follicles, promoting healthy growth. Think of it as a mini spa treatment you can do while binge-watching your favorite show. Another crucial step is gentle detangling. Use a wide-tooth comb or your fingers to remove knots, starting from the tips and working your way up. This prevents breakage and keeps your hair smooth and manageable.

Let's discuss a simple daily routine that can transform your hair game. In the morning, start with a light moisturizing spray. This helps to hydrate your hair and prep it for the day ahead. Look for products with natural ingredients like aloe vera or rose water for that extra boost. In the evening, switch to a silk or satin pillowcase. Unlike cotton, these materials reduce friction, preventing breakage and frizz while you sleep. Plus, they feel incredibly luxurious. It's a win-win.

Environmental factors can mess with your hair more than you might think. Wind can turn your hair into a tangled mess, while humidity makes it puff like a poodle's fur. On windy days, opt for protective hairstyles like braids or buns to keep your hair from turning into a bird's nest. For those humid days, use humidity-resistant products that help keep frizz at bay. These little adjustments can save you from a lot of hair drama.

Now, let's get into the must-have products for your daily routine. A good leave-in conditioner is a lifesaver. It keeps your hair moisturized throughout the day, making it easier to style and manage. Lightweight oils like Argan or Jojoba oil are also fantastic. They add shine without weighing your hair down, keeping it looking fresh and vibrant. A few drops can make a big difference, giving your hair that healthy, glossy finish.

Of course, not all hair is created equal, so it's essential to tailor your routine to your hair type. Light daily cleaning and volume-boosting products are your best friends if you have straight hair. They'll keep your hair looking sleek without making it flat. For wavy hair, leave-in conditioners and scrunching techniques help define those beautiful waves without making them crunchy. Curly hair thrives on daily hydration and curl-defining products. Look for creams and gels that enhance your natural curls while keeping them soft, coily hair benefits from rich creams and protective styling. Styles like twists or braids can help preserve moisture and keep your curls looking their best.

Building a healthy hair care routine doesn't have to be complicated. With the proper steps and products, you can achieve hair that looks and feels great. So give your hair the love it deserves, and watch it transform into the crowning glory you've always dreamed of.

2.2 Weekly Deep Conditioning: How And Why It's Important

Imagine your hair as a sponge left in the sun for too long. It's dry, brittle, and in desperate need of some TLC. This is where deep conditioning comes in. Think of it as a rejuvenating spa day for your hair. Deep conditioning treatments are like hydration bombs, intensely nourishing your hair and repairing damage caused by heat styling tools, environmental factors, and everyday wear and tear. Whether you're dealing with dryness, frizz, or damaged ends, an excellent deep conditioning session can breathe new life into your locks.

Selecting the right deep conditioner is crucial. Not all hair types have the exact needs, so knowing what works best for you can make a difference. A protein-based conditioner is your go-to if your hair feels weak. Protein helps to strengthen the hair shaft, making it more resilient. Conversely, opt for a moisture-rich conditioner if your hair is drier than the Sahara. These are packed with hydrating ingredients like shea butter or avocado oil and work wonders for restoring softness and shine. The key is to match the product to your hair's specific needs to get the best results.

So, how do you maintain a deep condition like a pro? Start by sectioning your hair. This ensures the product is evenly distributed, and every strand gets some love. Apply the conditioner generously, focusing on the mid-lengths and ends, where the hair is driest. For an extra boost, use a heat cap. The heat helps the conditioner penetrate deeper into the hair shaft, maximizing its benefits. Leave it on for the recommended time —usually about 20-30 minutes—then rinse thoroughly with cool water to seal the cuticle and lock in moisture. Voilà, you've just given your hair a mini makeover!

If you're a DIY enthusiast, you'll love making your own deep conditioning masks at home. One of my favorites is the avocado and honey mask. It's super easy to whip up and incredibly nourishing. Mash half an avocado and mix it with a tablespoon of honey. Apply it to your hair, leave it on for about 30 minutes, then rinse. Your hair will feel as soft as a cloud. Another great option is the coconut oil and yogurt mask. Combine a tablespoon of coconut oil with half a cup of yogurt. Coconut oil provides intense hydration, while yogurt protein strengthens your hair. Apply, leave on, and rinse—simple as that.

Deep conditioning is a game-changer for anyone looking to improve their hair health. It's not just about making your hair look good; it's about nourishing it from the inside out. Regular deep conditioning sessions can transform dry, brittle hair into soft, shiny, and resilient locks. Plus, it's a great way to pamper yourself and give your hair the attention it deserves. So treat your hair to a little spa day every week, and watch as it transforms from drab to fab.

2.3 Monthly Trims: Preventing Split Ends And Promoting Growth

Let's get honest about something that might seem counterintuitive—cutting your hair to make it grow. Trimming your hair regularly is like hitting the refresh button. It keeps your hair neat and prevents those dreaded split ends from traveling up the hair shaft. Imagine split ends as tiny invaders. If left unchecked, they can cause more damage, making your hair look frizzy and unhealthy. Regular trims help to stop them in their tracks, ensuring your hair stays strong and vibrant. Nobody wants to deal with scraggly ends that make styling a nightmare. Keeping your hair trimmed helps maintain a polished and tidy appearance, making you look put together even on your laziest days.

So, how often should you trim? It depends on your hair length and type. Aim for a trim every 4–6 weeks if you have short hair.

Short hair tends to lose shape quickly, and regular trims help keep it looking sharp. For those with longer locks, every 8–12 weeks is a good rule of thumb. Long hair doesn't need as frequent trims, but keeping those ends in check is still important. If you're trying to grow out your hair, you might be tempted to skip trims altogether. Resist the urge! Trimming a tiny bit every few months can actually help your hair grow healthier and prevent significant damage.

Now, if you're feeling brave and want to trim your hair at home, it's doable with the right tools and a steady hand. First off, invest in a pair of sharp, professional scissors. Kitchen scissors won't cut it—literally. Blunt blades can cause more harm than good, leading to more split ends and uneven cuts. When trimming, work in small sections. This gives you more control and helps ensure you don't accidentally chop off more than you intended. Start by trimming a small amount, about a quarter of an inch. You can always take off more if needed, but you can't return it once it's gone. Make sure to trim when your hair is dry to avoid any surprises. Wet hair looks longer, and you might cut more than you planned.

Recognizing when it is time for a trim is crucial. Keep an eye out for visible split ends. They're a clear sign that your hair needs some attention. Another clue is difficulty in styling. If your hair feels rough and unmanageable, it's probably time for a trim. Pay attention to how your hair behaves. If it's constantly getting tangled or feels unusually dry, a trim might be just what it needs. Regular trims help maintain your hair's health and make it easier to style, saving you time and frustration in the future.

Regular trims are a simple yet powerful tool in your hair care arsenal. They keep your hair fresh and healthy, prevent damage, and promote growth. Whether you are rocking a pixie cut or long, flowing locks, keeping up with trims is necessary, so grab those scissors or book an appointment with your stylist and give your hair the love it deserves.

2.4 Protecting Your Hair While You Sleep

Let's talk about something you probably never think about—what your hair does while you catch those Z's. Believe it or not, your hair can suffer a lot of damage while sleeping if you don't take the proper steps to protect it. Imagine tossing and turning all night, your hair rubbing against your pillow like it is auditioning for a sandpaper commercial. All that friction can lead to breakage and split ends, making your hair look less than fabulous. The key here is to minimize friction and balance your hair's moisture levels. It's like giving your hair a little night time spa treatment, ensuring it stays healthy and robust.

Adopting protective hairstyles is one of the easiest ways to protect your hair while you sleep. Loose braids or twists are fantastic options. They contain your hair and prevent it from tangling into a knotted mess. Plus, when you wake up, you can simply untwist or unbraid for some natural, heat-free waves. If you have curly hair, the pineapple method is a game-changer. Gather your hair into a high, loose ponytail on top of your head. This keeps your curls intact and prevents them from getting squished while you sleep. It's a simple trick that can make a huge difference in maintaining your curl pattern.

Now, let's get into the magic of silk and satin. If you're still using a cotton pillowcase, it's time to upgrade. Cotton can be rough on your hair, leading to frizz and breakage. Silk and satin, on the other hand, are much gentler. They reduce friction, helping to keep your hair smooth and frizz-free. Plus, they're better at maintaining your hairstyle. Whether you've got a fresh blowout or some killer curls, silk and satin pillowcases help preserve your style so you don't wake up with a hair disaster. And let's be honest, they feel luxurious. It's like giving your hair the VIP treatment it deserves.

Maintaining hair health overnight isn't just about what you sleep on; it's also about what you put in your hair before bed.

Applying a light oil before you hit the hay can work wonders. Think of it as a night cream for your hair. Oils like Argan or Jojoba help to lock in moisture, keeping your hair hydrated and shiny. Just a few drops go a long way, and you'll wake up with hair that feels soft and nourished. Another tip is to use a silk or satin bonnet. It's like a little sleeping bag protecting your hair from the elements. Plus, it helps to maintain your style, so you can wake up and go without much fuss.

Taking care of your hair while you sleep might seem like an extra step, but it pays off quickly. By reducing friction and keeping your hair hydrated, you're preventing damage and ensuring your hair stays healthy and robust. So, whether you braid, twist, or pineapple, give your hair some love before you hit the sack. And please don't forget that silk or satin pillowcase—it's a small investment with significant benefits.

2.5 Diy Hair Masks For Every Hair Type

Have you ever looked in your pantry and wondered if those bananas or that honey jar could do more than sit on your toast? Well, guess what? They can. DIY hair masks are a fantastic way to give your hair some much-needed TLC using natural ingredients you probably already have at home. The beauty of DIY masks is that you can customize them to suit your specific hair needs. No more guessing if that store-bought product is right for you. Plus, you avoid all the harsh chemicals that often lurk in commercial products. It's like giving your hair a fresh, organic smoothie instead of processed junk food.

Let's get into some recipes tailored for different hair types. If your hair is dry and desperately needs hydration, a banana and honey mask is your go-to. Bananas are packed with potassium and vitamins, which help to moisturize and strengthen your hair. Honey, on the other hand, is a natural humectant, meaning it locks in moisture. To make this mask:

1. Mix one ripe banana with two tablespoons of honey.
2. Apply the mixture evenly from roots to tips, ensuring every strand gets coated.
3. Leave it on for around 15–30 minutes, then rinse thoroughly with warm water. Your hair will feel like it just had a drink of water in a desert.

An egg and olive oil mask can work wonders for weak or brittle hair. Eggs are rich in protein, which helps to strengthen the hair shaft, while olive oil provides intense hydration and shine. To make this mask:

1. Beat one egg and mix it with two tablespoons of olive oil.
2. Apply it to your hair, focusing on the mid-lengths and ends where damage tends to be the worst.
3. Let it sit for around 15–20 minutes before rinsing with cool water. Trust me, your hair will thank you.

Now, let's talk about how to apply these masks properly. First, you want to make sure your ingredients are well-mixed. No one wants chunks of banana or egg whites stuck in their hair. Blend the ingredients until you get a smooth, creamy consistency. Once your mask is ready, apply it from the roots and work down to the tips. Use your fingers to massage the mask into your scalp and ensure even distribution. If you have a wide-tooth comb, it can help to spread the mask through your hair further. After applying, either wrap your hair in a warm towel or use a shower cap to keep the mask in place and add a bit of heat, which helps the ingredients penetrate better. Understanding the benefits of each ingredient can make your DIY hair mask even more effective. Honey is fantastic for moisture retention. It acts like a magnet, drawing moisture into your hair and keeping it there. Eggs are a powerhouse of protein and nutrients, helping to rebuild and strengthen your hair from the inside out. Olive oil is a natural emollient, providing deep conditioning and improving your hair's elasticity. Bananas are not just for smoothies; they offer vitamins and minerals that can make your hair softer and more manageable.

DIY hair masks are a fun and effective way to pamper your hair without breaking the bank. They allow you to tailor treatments to your specific needs, ensuring you get the best results. So, next time you're in the kitchen, look beyond your breakfast and consider how those ingredients can boost your hair. Whether you're battling dryness or weakness or want extra shine, there's a DIY mask for you.

2.6 The Role Of Diet And Nutrition In Hair Health

Let's get into something that's often overlooked but incredibly crucial—what you eat. Yes, your diet plays a massive role in the health of your hair. Think of your body as a factory and your food as raw materials. If you're not providing quality materials, the end product—your hair—won't be up to par. Nutrition influences everything from hair growth to strength. Essential nutrients are the building blocks for your hair, and deficiencies can lead to problems, from brittleness to hair loss.

Let's break down some essential nutrients that are absolute game-changers for hair health. Vitamin A is crucial for scalp health. It helps produce sebum, the natural oil that moisturizes your scalp and hair. Without enough vitamin A, your scalp can get dry and itchy, leading to weak hair. Zinc is another big player. It promotes hair growth and helps repair damaged hair follicles. Think of it as the handyman of your hair, fixing things up and ensuring everything runs smoothly. Omega-3 fatty acids are like the hydration superheroes. They keep your hair hydrated from the inside out, giving it that coveted shine and smooth texture.

So, what should you eat to get these nutrients? Leafy greens are a fantastic source of iron and vitamins. Spinach, kale, and Swiss chard are not just for salads; they're hair health powerhouses. Nuts and seeds are packed with healthy fats, proteins, and vitamins. Almonds, walnuts, and flaxseeds are great options to snack on or sprinkle over your meals. These foods are easy to incorporate into your diet and can make a significant difference in your hair's health.

Maintaining a balanced diet doesn't have to be complicated. One easy way to get a nutrient boost is through smoothies. Blend up some spinach, a banana, a handful of almonds, and a spoonful of flaxseeds with a splash of almond milk. Voilà, you've got a hair-boosting smoothie that tastes great and is packed with nutrients. Another tip is to plan your meals. Make sure each meal includes a good mix of protein, healthy fats, and veggies. This way, you're not just eating for your body but also for your hair.

Incorporating these nutrients into your daily diet can be a game-changer for your hair. You don't need to overhaul your entire eating plan; make minor adjustments and watch the magic happen. Your hair will become stronger, shinier, and more resilient, all thanks to the power of good nutrition. So, next time you plan a meal or grab a snack, think about how it can benefit your hair. It's a simple but effective way to give your hair the love it deserves.

To Summarize This Chapter:

Building a healthy hair care routine isn't as complicated as it might seem but requires dedication and consistency. Each step—from daily maintenance and deep conditioning to regular trims and mindful nighttime care—keeps your hair vibrant and resilient. And let's not overlook the impact of a balanced diet. Your hair is often a mirror of your overall health, so nourishing your body with the proper nutrients will help your hair radiate from the inside out.

Next, we'll explore the art of hair washing, delving into techniques and tips to ensure that every wash leaves your hair not just clean but also strong and happy!

CHAPTER 3: HAIR WASHING TECHNIQUES AND TIPS

So, let's dive into the nitty-gritty of washing your hair. Picture this: you're in the shower, belting out your favorite song, and you're not entirely sure if you're washing your hair the right way. Trust me, you're not alone. Washing your hair seems straightforward, but there's some science behind it. Let's clear up the confusion and get you on track to having clean, healthy hair without the guesswork.

3.1 How Often Should You Wash Your Hair?

First things first, how often should you wash your hair? The answer isn't one-size-fits-all. It depends on several factors, like your hair type, lifestyle, and scalp condition. Let's break it down. If you have an oily scalp, you might need to wash more frequently to keep that grease at bay. On the flip side, if your scalp is on the drier side, over-washing can strip it of the natural oils it desperately needs, leaving it parched and flaky.

Your lifestyle plays a significant role, too. If you hit the gym regularly or participate in sports, sweat buildup can make your hair feel dirty faster. In this case, more frequent washing might be necessary. Environmental factors like pollution and dust also come into play. Living in a bustling city with high pollution levels can make your hair feel grimy quickly, while a more rural setting might allow you to stretch the time between washes.

Now, let's get into some general guidelines for different hair types. If you have straight hair, aim to wash it every 2–3 days. Straight hair tends to get oily faster because natural oils can travel down the hair shaft more easily. For wavy hair, washing every 3–4 days is usually sufficient. Wavy hair strikes a balance between straight and curly, so it doesn't get as greasy as quickly but still needs regular cleansing. Curly hair can typically go a whole week between washes. The natural twists and turns of curly hair make it slower for oils to travel down the shaft, meaning it stays cleaner for longer. Coily hair, which is the most prone to dryness, can go as long as 1–2 weeks without washing. The tight coils make it even harder for natural oils to reach the ends, so washing your hair less often helps retain moisture.

But how do you know if you're over washing or underwashing? Overwashing can leave your hair dry and brittle, feeling like straw. It can also lead to an irritated scalp, which is no fun. On the other hand, under washing can make your hair greasy and weighed down, like you just dunked your head in a vat of oil. Finding that sweet spot is critical.

If you realize that you might be washing your hair too often, there are ways to adjust your routine gradually. Introducing dry shampoo can be a lifesaver. It helps absorb excess oil and gives your hair a fresh look without water. Try using it on the days between washes to extend the time between shampooing. Another trick is to use water-only rinses. This helps refresh your hair and scalp without stripping away those natural oils. Wet your hair, gently massage your scalp, and rinse thoroughly. It's a quick way to freshen up without the entire wash routine.

Understanding how often to wash your hair can make a huge difference in maintaining its health and appearance. By considering your hair type, lifestyle, and scalp condition, you can tailor your washing routine to fit your needs. So next time you're in the shower, you can confidently belt out that song, knowing your hair is getting the care it deserves.

3.2 Choosing The Right Shampoo And Conditioner For Your Hair Type

Let's get to the point: using the right shampoo and conditioner is like finding the perfect pair of jeans—they need to fit just right to make you feel fabulous. Mismatched products can lead to hair issues, from annoying buildup to dull, lifeless locks. When you nail the correct combo, your hair's natural texture and shine get a serious boost, making those good hair days a regular thing. It's not just about cleanliness; it's about enhancing what you've got and making it work for you.

Understanding your hair type's needs is the first step. Dry hair? You'll need a shampoo and conditioner packed with moisturizing ingredients like shea butter or coconut oil. These ingredients drench your hair in hydration, combating that dreaded dryness and brittleness. For fine hair, you'll want to volumize formulas. These products lift your strands from the roots without weighing them down, giving you that bouncy, complete look without the fluff. Damaged hair, whether from heat styling or chemical treatments, craves protein-rich products. Ingredients like keratin and silk proteins help rebuild the hair shaft, making it stronger and more resilient.

Now, let's get into some specific recommendations. A sulfate-free shampoo is your best bet if you've got color-treated hair. Sulfates can strip your color and leave your hair feeling like straw. For instance, **Olaplex No. 4 Bond Maintenance Shampoo** is a fantastic option. It's gentle and effective and works wonders for maintaining vibrant color. If you're battling an oily scalp, a clarifying shampoo like **Neutrogena's Anti-Residue Shampoo** can do the trick. It helps remove excess oil and product buildup without being too harsh. Curly hair folks, you'll love a deep conditioning treatment like **SheaMoisture's Jamaican Black Castor Oil Masque**. It provides intense moisture, making your curls pop with definition and shine.

Reading ingredient labels might seem like a chore, but it's crucial. You want to avoid sulfates and parabens like the plague. **Sulfates**, often listed as **sodium lauryl sulfate** or **sodium laureth sulfate**, can be too harsh, stripping your hair of its natural oils. **Parabens**, used as preservatives, can irritate your scalp and potentially mess with your hormones. Instead, look for natural oils and proteins. Ingredients like Argan oil, Jojoba oil, and hydrolyzed proteins are fantastic for nourishing and keeping your hair healthy. It's like feeding your hair a nutritious meal instead of junk food.

When choosing your products, think of it as a treasure hunt. You're searching for those gems that will make your hair look and feel amazing. Avoid falling for flashy marketing and focus on what's inside the bottle. A little bit of knowledge goes a long way in ensuring your hair gets the care it deserves. So, next time you're in the hair care aisle, take a moment to read those labels and choose wisely. Your hair will thank you, and you'll be strutting around with a healthy, shiny, and totally Instagram-worthy mane.

3.3 The Benefits Of Co-Washing And How To Do It Right

So, what's this buzz about co-washing you've probably seen all over social media? Co-washing, short for "conditioner-only washing," is a game-changer, especially for those with curly and coily hair. Instead of using shampoo, you use conditioner to cleanse your hair. Yes, you heard that right. This method helps retain your hair's natural oils, which shampoo often strips away, leaving your hair dry and brittle. Using conditioner instead keeps your hair hydrated and reduces the chances of breakage. It's like giving your hair a gentle hug instead of a harsh scrub.

The benefits of co-washing are numerous. For starters, it's fantastic for enhancing hydration. If you've got curls or coils, you know how much your hair craves moisture. Co-washing helps to lock in that much-needed hydration, making your hair softer and more manageable. It also reduces frizz. Imagine stepping out of the shower with hair that's smooth and defined, instead of looking like you've just stuck your finger in a socket. Another plus? Less breakage. By avoiding the harsh sulfates found in many shampoos, you're being kinder to your hair, which means fewer split ends and less breakage over time.

So, how do you co-wash like a pro? First, choose the right conditioner. Look for a lightweight, silicone-free option. Silicones can build up on your hair over time, making it feel heavy and greasy. You want something that cleanses without adding extra weight. Once you've picked your conditioner, get your hair thoroughly wet. Apply a generous amount of conditioner to your scalp and massage it in using your fingertips. This helps to lift dirt and oil from your scalp. Don't forget to distribute the conditioner evenly through the rest of your hair. After massaging for a few minutes, rinse thoroughly with lukewarm water. Make sure you get all the product out to avoid any residue.

Transitioning to co-washing can take a little time, but it's worth it. Start by alternating between co-washing and your regular shampoo routine to ease into it. This helps your scalp adjust slowly to the new method. Keep an eye on how your hair responds. If it starts to feel overly greasy, you might need to clarify with a gentle shampoo occasionally. On the flip side, if your hair feels great, you can co-wash it more frequently. It's all about finding that sweet spot where your hair feels clean and hydrated without being weighed down.

Co-washing can be a fantastic addition to your hair care routine, offering enhanced moisture, reduced frizz, and less breakage. It's particularly beneficial for curly and coily hair types that need all the hydration they can get. With the right conditioner and a bit of patience, you'll be on your way to softer, healthier hair. Give it a try and see how your hair responds. You might find it's the best thing you've ever done for your locks.

3.4 Avoiding Common Mistakes In Hair Washing

Let's discuss some common hair-washing blunders that can wreak havoc on your locks. First up, using hot water. Sure, a steaming hot shower feels incredible, but it's not doing your hair any favors. Hot water strips your scalp of natural oils, leaving your hair dry and brittle. It's like cooking your hair, and no one wants fried strands. Over-scrubbing the scalp is another biggie. While giving your scalp a vigorous scrub might seem like a good idea, it can cause irritation and even lead to hair thinning. Think of your scalp like delicate skin—it needs gentle care, not a rough scrub. And then there's the classic mistake of applying conditioner to the roots. This might seem harmless, but it's a surefire way to end up with greasy, weighed-down hair. Conditioner is meant to hydrate the ends, not the scalp.

Now, let's break down the consequences of these mistakes. When you use hot water, you're essentially drying out your hair. This leads to dull, lifeless locks that are prone to breakage. Imagine your hair snapping like dry spaghetti—ouch! Over-scrubbing your scalp can cause redness, irritation, and even hair loss over time. It's like taking sandpaper to your scalp; trust me, that's not a good look. Applying conditioner to the roots can leave your hair feeling greasy and heavy. It's like putting lotion on your face and then wondering why you're breaking out. Your scalp produces enough oil on its own; it doesn't need extra help from the conditioner.

So, what's the fix? First, switch to lukewarm or cool water to rinse your hair. It might not be as cozy as hot water, but your hair will thank you. Cool water helps to close the hair cuticle, making your hair look shinier and smoother. Plus, it's way better for retaining moisture. When washing your hair, gently massage your scalp with your fingertips instead of scrubbing it like you're trying to remove a stubborn stain. This helps to stimulate blood flow without causing damage. And when it comes to conditioner, apply it only to the mid-lengths and ends of your hair. These are the areas that need the most moisture, not your roots.

Proper rinsing is another crucial step that often gets overlooked. Leaving even a tiny bit of shampoo or conditioner in your hair can lead to product buildup, making your hair look greasy and dull. It's like leaving soap on your skin—gross, right? Make sure to rinse your hair thoroughly until the water runs clear. This ensures that no residue is left behind, leaving your hair feeling fresh and clean.

Avoiding these common hair-washing mistakes can make a world of difference in your hair's health and appearance. By making a few simple changes, you can keep your hair looking its best and avoid the pitfalls of improper washing techniques. So next time you're in the shower, remember these tips and give your hair the love and care it deserves.

3.5 The "No-Poo" Method: Is It Right For You?

Have you ever heard of the "No-Poo" method and thought, "What in the world is that?" Well, let me break it down for you. The No-Poo method is about ditching traditional shampoos and embracing a more natural approach to hair care. Instead of using shampoo, you cleanse your hair with baking soda and condition it with apple cider vinegar. Yup, those kitchen staples aren't just for baking and salad dressing anymore. The philosophy behind No-Poo is to reduce the exposure to harsh chemicals found in many commercial shampoos. This method emphasizes natural hair care, aiming to let your hair maintain its natural oils and balance.

So, what are the potential benefits of going No-Poo? For starters, you'll reduce exposure to harsh chemicals that can strip your hair of its natural oils. Many shampoos contain sulfates and parabens, which can lead to dry, brittle hair. By avoiding these, you give your hair a chance to thrive naturally. Another perk is balanced scalp oil production. When you stop stripping your scalp of its natural oils, it learns to regulate itself better. This means less greasy roots and more balanced, healthy hair. Many people find their hair softer, shinier, and more manageable over time. It's like letting your hair go on a health retreat.

How do you do this No-Poo thing? It's pretty simple. Start

by mixing one tablespoon of baking soda with one cup of water. This mixture acts as your cleanser. Pour it over your wet hair and massage it into your scalp, just like you would with regular shampoo. Rinse thoroughly with water. Next, mix one to two tablespoons of apple cider vinegar with one cup of water. This will be your conditioner. Pour it over your hair, focusing on the mid-lengths and ends. Let it sit for a few minutes, then rinse with cool water. The vinegar helps to smooth the hair cuticle and add shine. Now, here's the kicker: there's a transition period. Your hair might feel greasy or waxy for the first few weeks as it adjusts to the new routine. Don't freak out! This is normal and part of the process.

Are you wondering if No-Poo is right for you? It's not a one-size-fits-all solution and might not work for everyone. Start by monitoring how your hair and scalp respond. If your hair feels heavy or greasy, you might need to adjust the ratios of baking soda and vinegar or rinse more thoroughly. Pay attention to your scalp as well. The method might not be for you if it becomes itchy or irritated. On the flip side, if your hair starts to feel softer and your scalp balances out, you're on the right track. You can also adjust the frequency of your No-Poo routine based on your hair's needs. Some people only need to cleanse their hair once a week, while others might do it more frequently. It's all about finding what works best for you.

The No-Poo method can be a fantastic way to improve your hair health naturally. You could see some impressive results by reducing exposure to harsh chemicals and allowing your scalp to regulate its oil production. Plus, you're using ingredients that are cheap and easily accessible. It's a win-win! Give it a try and see how your hair responds. You might be surprised at how much healthier and happier your locks become.

3.6 How To Properly Detangle Hair Without Damage

Detangling might seem like a mundane task, but doing it

wrong can lead to a hair catastrophe. Imagine spending months growing out your hair, only to end up with split ends and breakage because you rushed through detangling. Incorrect detangling can cause severe damage, leading to split ends and hair loss. This is because yanking through knots can snap your hair, making it more prone to split ends. Consistently breaking your hair can also mess up its length and integrity. Over time, this leaves you with uneven, damaged hair that's a nightmare to style.

Different hair types require different detangling techniques. A regular brush works fine for straight hair, but you still need to be gentle. Wavy hair benefits from a detangling brush that can glide through the waves without snagging. Curly hair? That's where a wide-tooth comb comes in. It's perfect for gently working through those curls without causing breakage. Coily hair, on the other hand, thrives with finger detangling. Your fingers are less likely to cause breakage and can feel out knots more delicately. Each hair type has its own quirks; recognizing them helps you choose the best detangling method.

When it comes to tools, not all are created equal. Wide-tooth combs are fantastic for all hair types, especially curly and coily hair. They help to detangle without pulling or breaking the hair. Like the Tangle Teezer, detangling brushes are designed to glide through knots effortlessly, making them ideal for wavy and curly hair. Leave-in conditioners and detangling sprays are lifesavers. They add slip to your hair, making it easier to detangle without causing damage. These products coat your hair, reducing friction and making it easier to comb through.

So, how do you detangle your hair without turning it into a frizzy mess? Start by applying a detangler or leave-in conditioner to damp hair. This gives your hair some much-needed slip, making it easier to work through. Divide your hair into manageable sections. This allows you to focus on one area at a time, reducing the risk of breakage. Begin detangling from the ends of your hair, working your way up to the roots. This method minimizes tugging and reduces the chances of snapping your hair. Use gentle, slow strokes, and if you hit a knot, don't yank. Instead, work the knot out gently with your fingers or a wide-tooth comb.

Proper detangling is crucial for maintaining healthy hair. It prevents split ends, reduces breakage, and helps keep your hair looking its best. Using the correct techniques and tools, you can detangle your hair safely and effectively, preserving its length and integrity. So, next time you're faced with a head full of tangles, remember these tips and give your hair the gentle care it deserves.

Wrapping Up Chapter Three

Understanding how to wash and detangle your hair can significantly enhance its health and overall appearance. By tailoring your routine to your specific hair type and needs, you can keep your locks looking fabulous every day. Next, we'll explore different styling techniques that will help you rock any look effortlessly.

CHAPTER 4: STYLING TECHNIQUES FOR BEGINNERS

Have you ever stared at a YouTube tutorial and wondered if you need a degree in engineering to recreate that hairstyle? We've all been there. The good news is that styling your hair doesn't have to be complicated. With the right tools and a little practice, you can achieve salon-worthy looks right at home. Let's dive into the essentials that will transform your hair game from "meh" to "wow."

4.1 Tools Of The Trade: Brushes, Combs, And More

First things first, let's talk about the unsung heroes of hairstyling—your brushes and combs. These tools can make or break your styling efforts, so knowing which ones to use is crucial. Paddle brushes are your go-to for detangling and smoothing. With their broad, flat base, they glide through your hair like a dream, tackling knots without causing breakage. If you're aiming for volume and curls, round brushes are your best friend. They work wonders when blow-drying, helping to lift the roots and create those bouncy curls you've always wanted.

Wide-tooth combs are perfect for detangling wet hair. They're gentle and reduce the risk of breakage, making them ideal for curly and thick hair types. On the other hand, fine-tooth combs are all about precision. Whether you're parting your hair or smoothing out flyaways, these combs give you the control you need for detailed work.

Choosing the right tool depends on your hair type. If you have fine hair, natural bristle brushes are your best bet. They're gentle and help distribute your hair's natural oils, giving your hair a healthy shine. Boar bristle brushes are excellent for all hair types but especially for distributing natural oils from roots to ends. Metal combs can help manage the volume without causing damage if your hair is thick or coarse. They're sturdy and can handle the extra resistance that comes with thicker hair strands.

Keeping your tools in top condition is just as important as choosing the right ones. Regular cleaning is a must. Remove hair and debris after each use to keep your brushes and combs effective. For a deeper clean, soak them in warm water mixed with a bit of shampoo. This helps remove any product buildup and keeps your tools hygienic. When it comes to storage, avoid damp environments. Moisture can cause mold and mildew, which is a big no-no for anything you're putting on your hair. Store your tools in a dry, ventilated area to keep them fresh and ready for action.

Beyond the basics, every beginner should have a few additional tools in their arsenal. Hair ties and elastics are essential for securing styles. Go for ones that are gentle on your hair to avoid breakage. Hair clips and sectioning tools are lifesavers when you're working on more intricate styles. They help keep your hair organized and make the styling process much smoother. Clips are also great for holding curls in place while they set, giving you a longer-lasting volume.

The right tools can make a world of difference in your styling routine. Whether you're detangling, adding volume, or creating intricate styles, having the proper brushes and combs is critical. Keep them clean and well-maintained, and they'll serve you well for years to come. So next time you're struggling with a style, take a step back and check your tools—you might need a little upgrade.

4.2 Mastering The Basic Ponytail And Variations

Let's get into one of the most versatile and classic hairstyles —the ponytail. It's a go-to for a reason, because it's simple, quick, and can be dressed up or down.
To start, gather your hair at the desired height. Whether you're going for a high, mid, or low ponytail, make sure you've brushed through any tangles for a smooth finish. Once your hair is gathered, secure it with a hair tie. Here's a pro tip: use a strong, snag-free elastic to avoid hair breakage. For added hold, give your ponytail a light spritz of hairspray. This helps keep stray hairs in place and adds a bit of shine. After securing, take a moment to smooth out any bumps. You can use a brush or your fingers to gently even out the hair. Voilà! You've got yourself a classic ponytail.

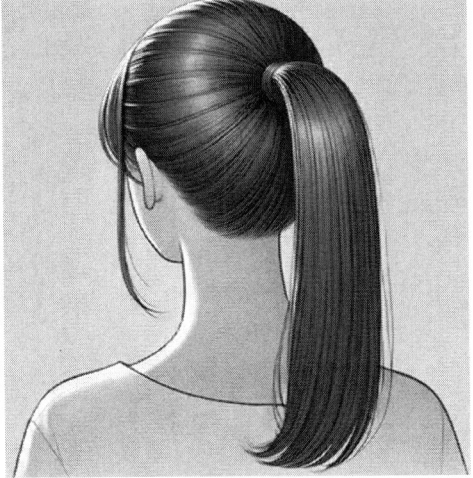

But why stop at basic when you can elevate your ponytail game with a few variations? A high ponytail gives you a sleek, polished look. It's perfect for when you want to look chic but don't have a lot of time. Simply gather your hair at the crown of your head and secure it tightly. On the other hand, a low ponytail offers a more laid-back, casual vibe. Gather your hair at the nape of your neck and secure it loosely for a relaxed look. The side ponytail is your friend for those who like a bit of asymmetry. Gather your hair to one side and secure it just below your ear for a playful, youthful style.

Want to make your ponytail look more polished and voluminous? Try wrapping a strand of hair around the hair tie. This little trick hides the elastic and adds a touch of elegance. Simply take a small section of hair from the ponytail, wrap it around the base, and secure it with a bobby pin. Another way to amp up your ponytail is by teasing the crown. Use a fine-tooth comb to gently backcomb the hair at the crown before gathering it into a ponytail. This adds volume and gives your ponytail a more lifted, glamorous look.

Accessories can also take your ponytail from basic to fabulous. Decorative hair ties are an easy way to add some pizzazz. Look for ones with embellishments like pearls or rhinestones. Hair scarves and ribbons are another fun option. Tie a colorful scarf or ribbon around your ponytail for a boho-chic look. Statement clips can also add a bit of flair. Place a clip at the base of your ponytail or along the side to draw attention and make your style stand out.

So there you have it! The ponytail isn't just a fallback option; it's a versatile style that can be as simple or intricate as you want it to be. With these tips and variations, you'll never have to worry about a boring ponytail again.

4.3 Easy Braiding Techniques: From Three-Strand To Waterfall

Let's start with the bread and butter of braiding—the three-strand braid. Add photo series. This is the foundation for so many styles, and once you get the hang of it, the sky's the limit!

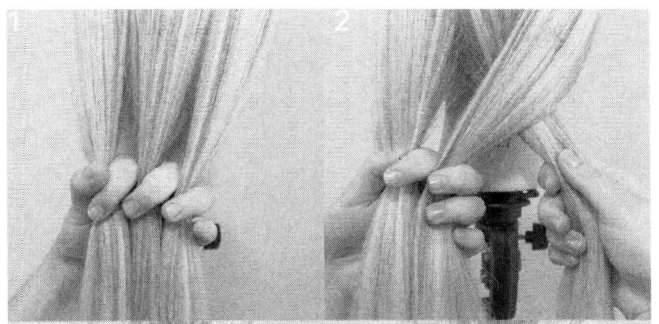

First, make sure your hair is smooth and tangle-free. Divide your hair into three equal sections. Hold two sections in one hand and the third in the other. Start by crossing the right section over the middle section.

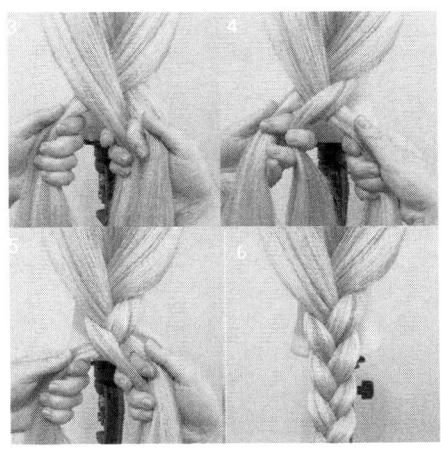

Then, take the left section and cross it over the new middle section. Continue this pattern, alternating right and left sections over the middle until you reach the ends of your hair. Secure the braid with a hair tie, and you've got yourself a classic three-strand braid. Easy, right?

Next up is the fishtail braid. This one looks intricate but is actually simple once you get the hang of it.

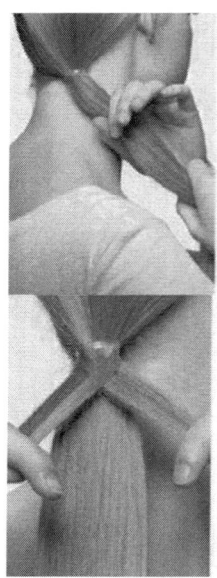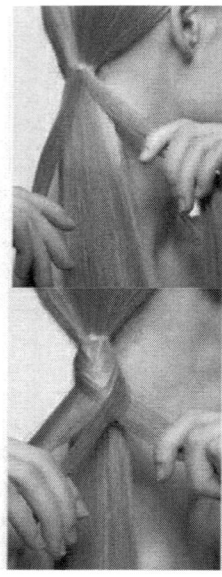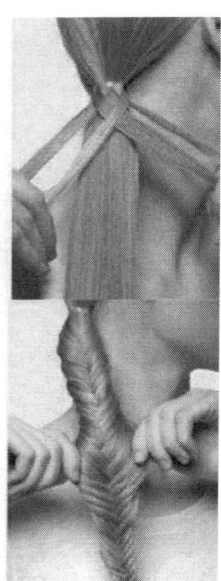

Begin by dividing your hair into two equal sections. Take a small piece of hair from the outer edge of the left section and cross it over to the right section. Then, take a small piece from the outer edge of the right section and cross it over to the left section. Repeat this process, alternating sides, until you reach the end of your hair. Secure with a small elastic, and you've got a stunning fishtail braid that's sure to impress.

Let's get a bit fancy with the waterfall braid. This style is perfect for adding a touch of elegance to your look.

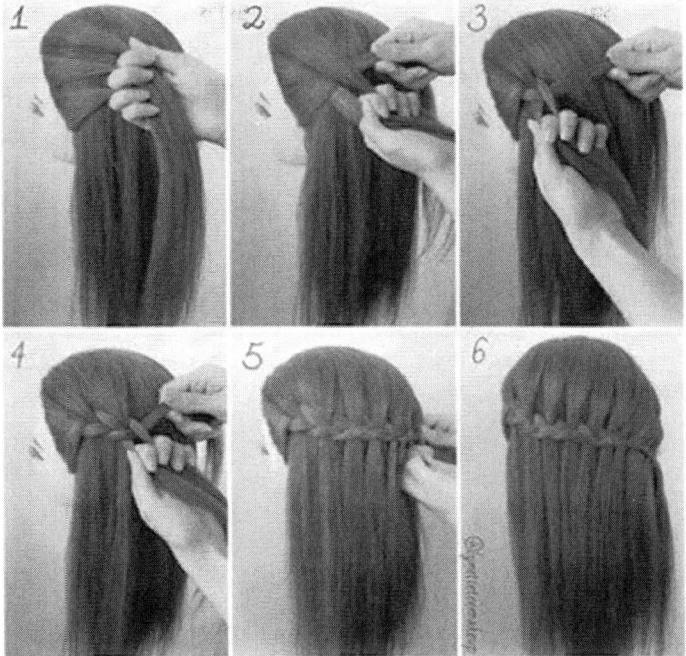

- Start by taking a section of hair from the front and dividing it into three smaller sections.
- Begin a three-strand braid, but drop the hair's bottom section after the first crossover.
- Pick up a new section of hair just behind the dropped piece and continue braiding. Each time you drop a section, pick up a new one to add to the braid. This creates the beautiful "waterfall" effect. Secure the braid with a hair tie or blend it into a traditional braid to finish the look.

Let's get a bit fancy with the waterfall braid. This style is perfect for adding a touch of elegance to your look. Start by taking a section of hair from the front and dividing it into three smaller sections. Begin a three-strand braid, but drop the hair's bottom section after the first crossover. Pick up a new section of hair just behind the dropped piece and continue braiding. Each time you drop a section, pick up a new one to add to the braid. This creates the beautiful "waterfall" effect. Secure the braid with a hair tie or blend it into a traditional braid to finish the look.

Here are a few tips to perfect your braids and keep them looking fresh all day: Use a bit of styling gel or mousse to hold it. This helps control any flyaways and adds grip to your hair, making it easier to braid. For a fuller, more relaxed look, gently pull apart the braid after securing it. This adds volume and gives your braid a softer appearance. Finally, make sure to secure the ends tightly with a small elastic to keep everything in place.

Braiding might seem daunting at first, but with a bit of practice, you'll be able to create a variety of stunning styles. Whether heading to school, work, or a special event, these braids will make you look fabulous and feel confident.

4.4 Creating Quick And Stylish Buns

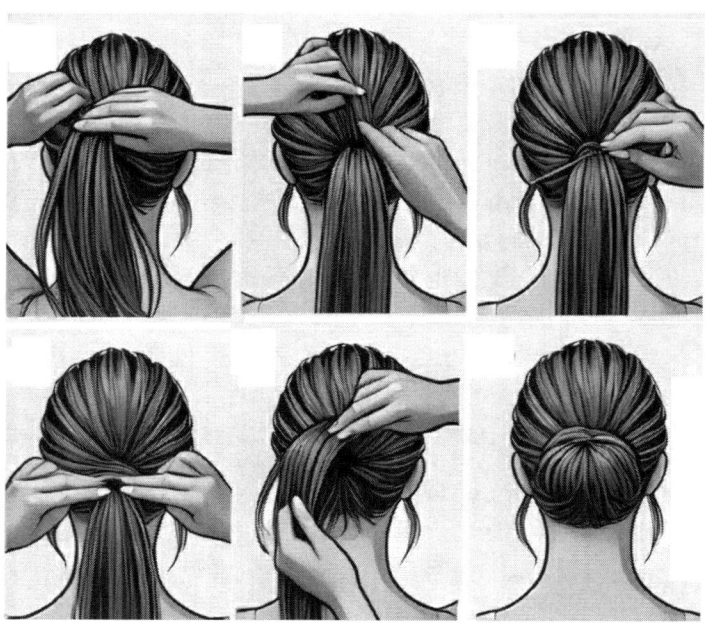

- Let's start with the classic bun, your go-to for a sleek,

polished look that works for any occasion—from a day at school to a night out.
- First, gather your hair into a ponytail at your desired height: high for a chic look, mid-level for everyday wear, or low for a more relaxed vibe.
- Once your ponytail is secured with a hair tie, twist the ponytail into a coil.
  - Think of it like twisting a rope. Now, wrap that coil around the base of your ponytail to form a bun.

Secure it with a few bobby pins, making sure to tuck in any loose ends. And just like that, you've got a classic bun that holds up all day.

Let's talk about the messy bun, the ultimate in laid-back cool. This style is perfect for those days when you want to look effortlessly stylish without putting in a ton of effort.

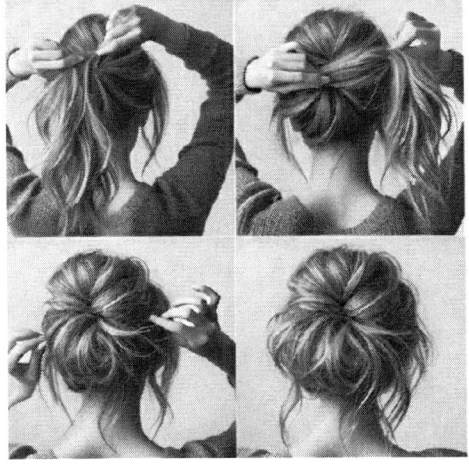

- Start by loosely gathering your hair into a high ponytail. Don't worry about making it perfect; the whole point is to keep it relaxed.
- Twist the ponytail and secure it with a hair tie.
- The magic happens here: pull out a few strands around your face and the nape of your neck to create that messy, undone effect.
- You can even tug on the bun a bit to make it look fuller

and more casual.

Ever wondered how people get those perfect round buns that look like they belong on a ballerina? Enter the sock bun technique.

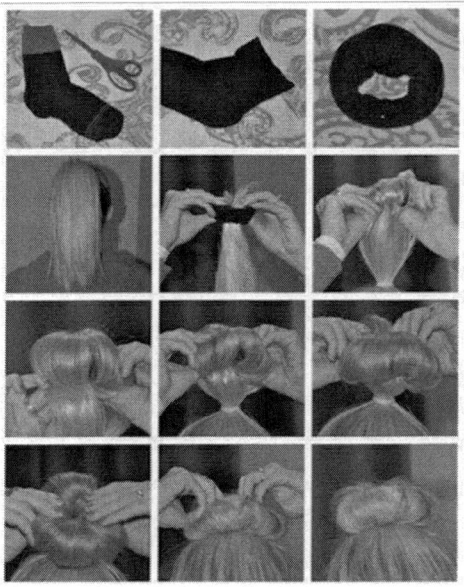

- Grab an old sock and cut off the toe, then roll it into a doughnut shape.
- Pull your ponytail through the donut's center and spread your hair evenly around it.
- Now, start rolling the sock down, tucking your hair under as you go.
- Keep rolling until you reach the base of your ponytail.

Secure it with a few bobby pins, and you've got a flawless, round bun that looks like you spent hours on it.
Please don't underestimate the power of accessories when it comes to buns. Decorative hair pins can add a touch of elegance to a simple bun. Slide in a few pins around the base of your bun for a bit of sparkle. If you're feeling boho, wrap a colorful scarf

around your bun. It's a quick way to add flair and personality to your look. Headbands are another versatile accessory. Choose a sleek, metallic headband for a sophisticated look or a fabric one for something more casual.

Buns aren't one-size-fits-all, and different hair lengths call for other techniques. If you've got short hair, bobby pins are your best friend. Use them liberally to secure your bun and keep those shorter strands in place. For medium-length hair, aim for a balanced bun that's not too tight or too loose. This length gives you the perfect amount of hair to create a whole, voluminous bun without a lot of effort. Long hair offers the most versatility. You can wrap and tuck your hair in various ways to create intricate bun styles. Don't be afraid to experiment with different wrapping techniques to find what works best for you.

And there you have it—quick and stylish buns that are easy to master and perfect for any occasion. Whether you're going for a polished look or something more casual, these bun techniques have got you covered.

4.5 Everyday Hairstyles For School And Work

Life can get pretty hectic, and the last thing you need is to spend an hour wrestling with your hair every morning. That's why practical hairstyles are a lifesaver. They save you precious time, ensure you look professional, and keep you comfortable throughout the day. Imagine trying to focus on a math test or a work presentation while constantly adjusting your hair. Not fun, right? Practical styles help you avoid that hassle, making your day smoother and more efficient.

If you're looking for something versatile, the half-up, half-down style is your best bet. It's the perfect blend of casual and formal, making it suitable for almost any occasion.

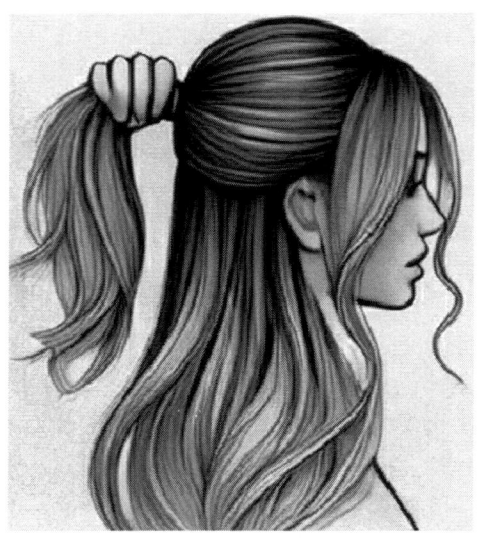

- Start by sectioning off the top half of your hair. You can use a comb to create a clean part or go for a more relaxed, messy look.
- Secure the top half with a clip or hair tie. Now, here's where you can get creative: add some curls or waves to the loose hair for extra volume and texture. Use a curling iron or braid your hair overnight for natural waves. This style is effortlessly chic and works well with all hair types.

If you want something a bit more polished, the sleek low bun is your answer.

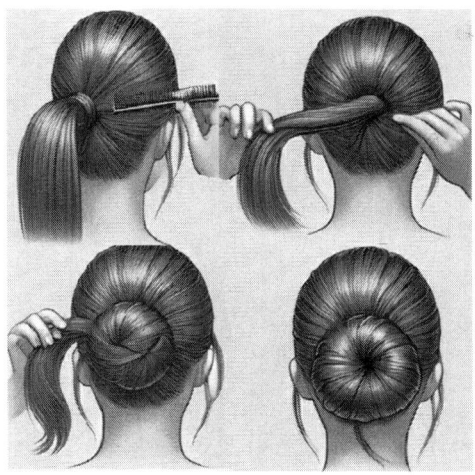

- Start by gathering your hair at the nape of your neck.
- Smooth it down with a brush to get rid of any bumps.
- Once you've got a smooth base, twist your hair into a bun and secure it with bobby pins.
- To achieve that sleek finish, apply a bit of gel to smooth down any flyaways. This style looks professional and stays put throughout the day, making it ideal for busy schedules.

Braids are another fantastic option for those hectic mornings. They look intricate but are surprisingly easy to do. A side braid is a quick and stylish choice. Simply gather your hair to one side, divide it into three sections, and start braiding. Secure it with a hair tie, and you're good to go.

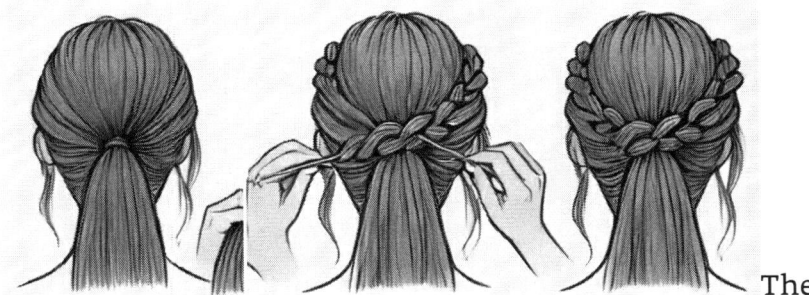

The braided headband is another fun style. Take a small section of hair from behind your ear, braid it, and then wrap it across the top of your head like a headband. Secure it with a bobby pin on the other side. It's a cute and practical way to keep your hair out of your face.

Practical hairstyles are essential for making your daily routine more manageable. They save you time, keep you looking professional, and ensure you are comfortable all day long. Whether you opt for a ponytail, a sleek bun, or a quick braid, these styles have got you covered. So next time you're rushing to get ready, remember these easy, practical hairstyles and step out the door with confidence.

4.6 Heatless Curls And Waves: Methods And Benefits

Let's talk about getting those luscious curls without frying your hair in the process. Heatless curls are a fantastic way to keep your hair healthy while still achieving that dreamy, wavy look. One of the biggest perks of avoiding heat is reducing damage. Heat styling tools can wreak havoc on your hair, leading to dryness, split ends, and breakage. Opting for heatless methods maintains your hair's natural moisture levels, keeping it soft and shiny. Plus, you're preventing those pesky split ends that make your hair look frizzy and unkempt.

So, how do you get those gorgeous curls without a curling iron? One popular method is the twist-and-wrap technique. Add photo series. Start by dividing your hair into sections. The number of sections depends on how tight you want your curls to be. For tighter curls, create more sections; for looser waves, go with fewer. Take each section and twist it tightly from root to tip. Once twisted, wrap the section around itself to form a mini bun and secure it with a clip. Do this for all sections and leave them overnight. When you wake up, gently unwrap the twists, and voilà! You've got beautiful curls without the heat damage.

Another great way to achieve waves is by braiding your hair before bed. Start with damp hair for the best results. Divide your hair into multiple sections and create braids. The more braids you do, the tighter the waves will be. Sleep with the braids in place and unravel them in the morning. You'll be left with natural-looking waves that look effortlessly chic. This method is incredibly excellent for those with longer hair, as it helps reduce frizz and keeps your hair looking polished.

To make your heatless curls last longer and look more defined, you can use a few handy tricks. First, apply a light mousse or curl-enhancing product to your hair before starting the twist or braid process. This helps to hold the shape and adds some extra definition to your curls. Once you've achieved your curls, scrunch them gently to add volume and enhance their natural shape. Be careful not to brush out the curls, as this can lead to frizz and ruin all your hard work. Instead, use your fingers to separate and style the curls for a more natural look.

Heatless curls are a fantastic way to keep your hair healthy while still looking fabulous. Whether you're using the twist-and-wrap method or braiding your hair for waves, these techniques are easy to master and perfect for any hair type. Plus, you'll be saving your hair from the damage that comes with heat styling, keeping it soft, shiny, and full of life. So next time you want to rock those curls, give these heatless methods a try and see how amazing your hair can look without the heat.

CHAPTER 5: ADVANCED STYLING TECHNIQUES

Ever found yourself scrolling through Instagram, mesmerized by those intricate braids and wondering if you could ever pull them off? Trust me, I've been there. Let's take a deep breath and dive into the wonderful world of advanced styling techniques. This chapter is all about taking your hair game to the next level with some seriously cool braiding techniques. Ready to become a braid master? Let's get started.

5.1 The Art Of French Braiding And Dutch Braiding

First up, let's tackle the French braid. This classic style is both elegant and practical, perfect for keeping your hair out of your face while looking effortlessly chic.

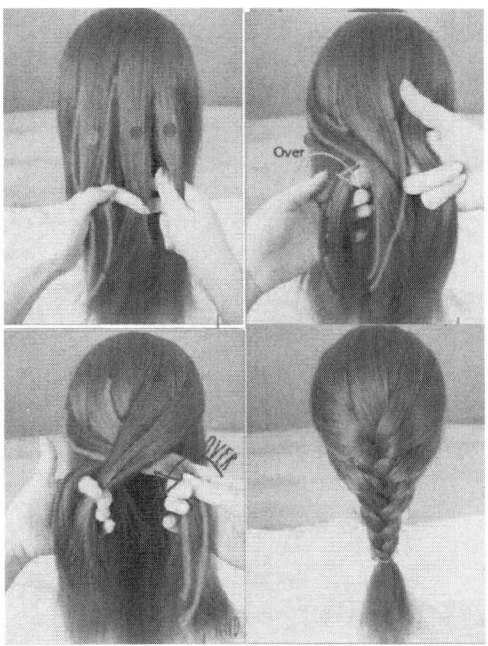

- Start by brushing your hair to remove any tangles. Now, gather a section of hair from the top center of your head. This is your starting point, so make sure it's a decent-sized chunk. Divide this section into three equal parts.
- Here's where the magic begins: start with a traditional braid by crossing the right strand over to the center, then the left strand over to the center. Got it? Good.
- Now, before you make the next crossover, add a small piece of hair from the side of your head to the outer section you're about to cross over.
- Continue this process, adding new sections of hair each time you cross a strand over. Keep braiding until you've incorporated all your hair.
- At this point, you can either secure the braid at the nape of your neck or continue braiding down to the ends. Secure with a hair tie, and voilà, you've got yourself a beautiful French braid.

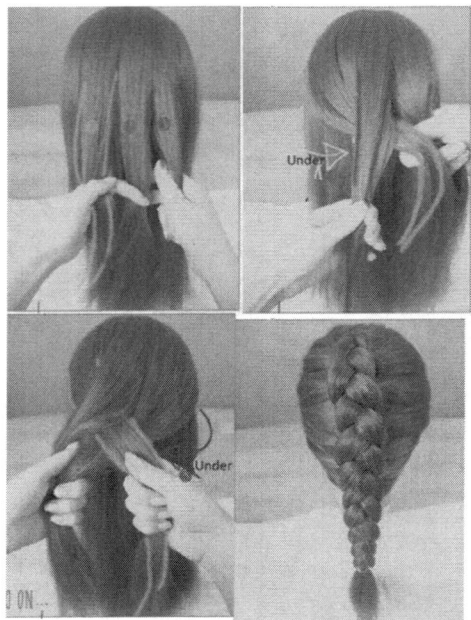

Now, let's switch things up with the Dutch braid. Think of it as the French braid's edgy cousin. The main difference here is that instead of crossing the strands over the middle, you'll be crossing them under. This creates a more pronounced, three-dimensional braid that really stands out.

- Start by gathering a section of hair from the crown of your head and dividing it into three parts.
- Begin by crossing the right strand under the middle strand, then the left strand under the middle strand. Just like with the French braid, add small sections of hair to the outer strands before crossing them under the middle. Continue this process, making sure to keep the sections tight for a neat look. Once all your hair is included, finish with a traditional braid and secure it with a hair tie. The result? A stunning Dutch braid that's sure to turn heads.

Perfecting these braids takes a bit of practice, but don't get

discouraged. For a more polished look, keep the sections tight and even. This helps to create a neat, professional finish. If you're struggling to keep the hair in place, try braiding on damp hair. The added moisture gives you better grip and control, making it easier to manage. Another tip is to use small hair clips to hold sections in place as you braid. This can be especially helpful when you're just starting out and need a bit of extra help.
Once you've got the hang of the basics, it's time to get creative with variations and style.

Double Dutch braids are perfect for a sporty look.

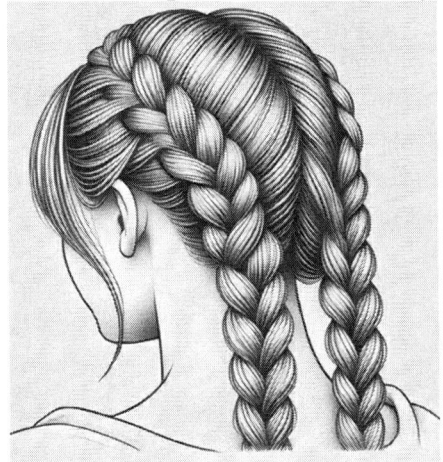

- Simply create two Dutch braids on either side of your head,
- Starting at the crown and working your way down. This style is not only practical but also super cute.

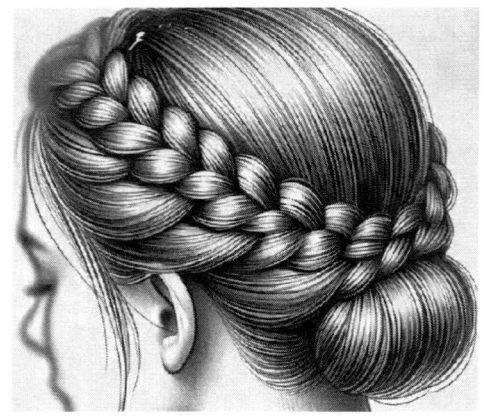

For a more romantic vibe, try a French braid crown.

- Start braiding from one side of your head, working your way around the back, and ending on the other side.
- Secure the braid with bobby pins, and you've got a gorgeous, fairy-tale-worthy look.

A side-swept French braid is your best bet you're going for something more casual.

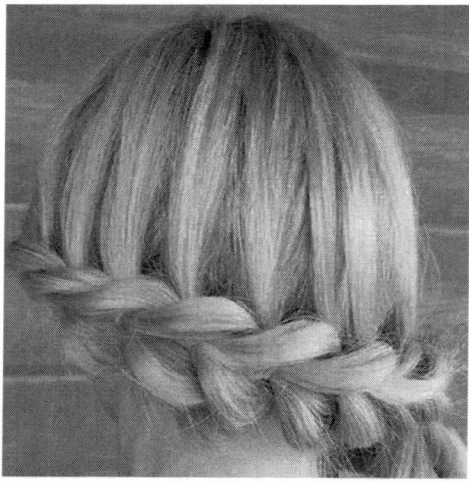

- Start the braid at the crown and work your way down one side, securing the end with a hair tie. It's laid-back yet stylish, perfect for a day out with friends.

And that leads me to the French braid ponytail, start with a French braid at the crown of your head and transition into a ponytail once you reach the nape. Secure with an elastic, and you've got a stylish yet functional hairstyle.

Braiding might seem daunting at first, but with patience and practice, you'll be amazed at what you can achieve. So grab a mirror, take a deep breath, and start braiding. Your hair is your canvas, and the possibilities are endless.

5.2 Creating Elegant Chignons And Twists

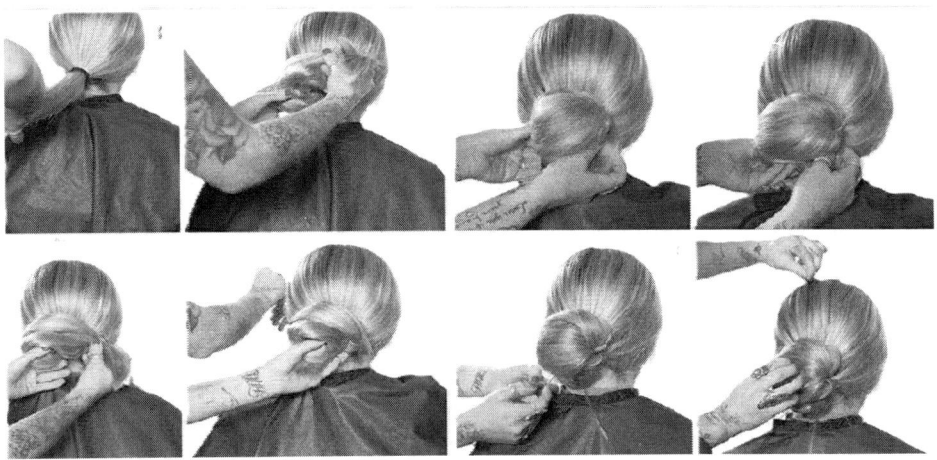

Let's break down the classic chignon, a timeless style that screams elegance.

- Start by gathering your hair into a low ponytail at the nape of your neck.
- Make sure it's smooth and tangle-free.
- Once your ponytail is secured with a hair tie, twist the ponytail tightly. Think of it like winding up a rope.
- Coil the twisted ponytail around the base, forming a neat bun. Secure it with bobby pins, making sure to tuck

in any loose ends. A spritz of hairspray will help keep everything in place, giving you a sleek, polished look perfect for any fancy occasion.

Now, let's up the ante with a twisted chignon.

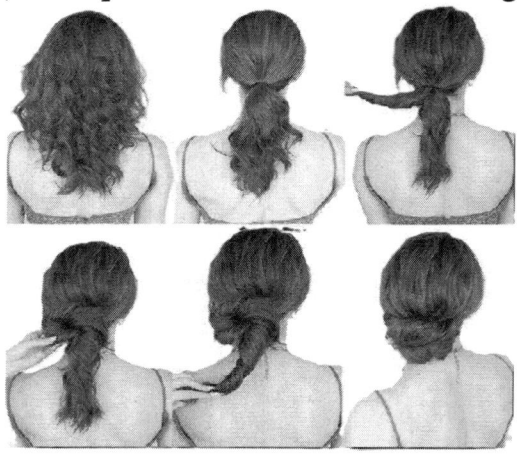

- This style is a bit more intricate but totally worth the effort. Start by dividing your hair into several sections. The number of sections depends on how textured you want the final look to be.
- Take each section and twist it tightly, just like you did with the basic chignon. Once twisted, coil each section around the base of your ponytail, pinning as you go. This creates a layered, textured look that adds depth and dimension to your chignon.
- Secure everything with bobby pins and finish with hairspray to lock in the style. This twisted variation looks incredibly sophisticated and is perfect for weddings, proms, or any event where you want to feel extra special.

Next, let's dive into the rope twist technique, a fantastic way to create elegant updos.

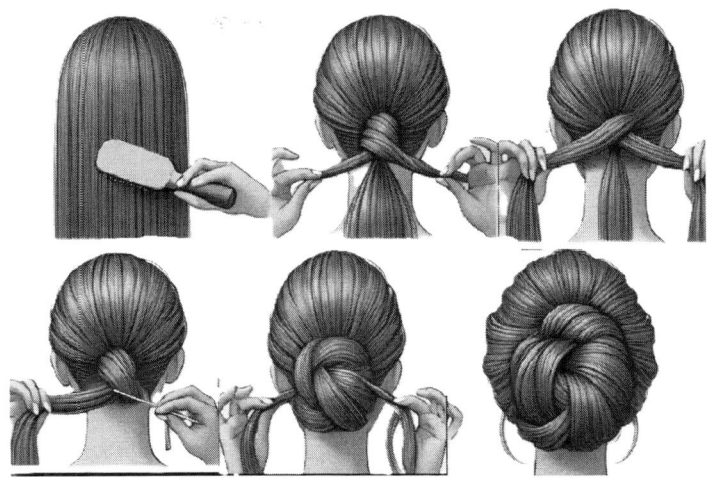

- Start by dividing your hair into two equal sections.
- Take one section and twist it tightly from root to tip.
- Now, do the same with the other section. Once both sections are twisted, twist them around each other like you're braiding a rope. Secure the end with a small elastic.
- You can then coil the twisted rope around the base of your ponytail or pin it up in various ways to create different updo styles. The rope twist is versatile and can be dressed up or down depending on the occasion.

Intricate updos, like chignons, are ideal for more formal events. Add photo series. Start by sectioning your hair and creating a low ponytail. Twist the ponytail into a coil and secure it with bobby pins. You can then add braids or twists to the remaining hair, wrapping them around the base of the chignon for added detail. Finish with hairspray and a few decorative pins, and you're ready to go. This style is both elegant and sophisticated, perfect for a night when you want to feel like royalty.

To make sure your chignons and twists last all day (or night), there are a few tips you'll want to keep in mind. First, always start with hair that has a bit of texture. Clean, slippery hair can be challenging to manage and may also not hold the style. A bit of dry shampoo or texturizing spray can give you the grip you need. When securing your chignon or twists, use plenty of bobby pins. Don't be shy; you want to make sure everything stays put. For extra hold, crisscross the bobby pins. This creates a stronger anchor and helps keep the style secure. Finally, finish with a good dose of hairspray. Not only does it help hold the style, but it also tames any flyaways and adds a bit of shine.

Chignons and twists are timeless styles that can elevate any look. Whether you're going for a classic, sleek chignon or a more intricate, twisted version, these styles are sure to make you feel elegant and polished. With a bit of practice and the proper techniques, you'll be able to create these beautiful updos with ease. So grab those bobby pins, twist away, and get ready to turn heads with your stunning hairstyle.

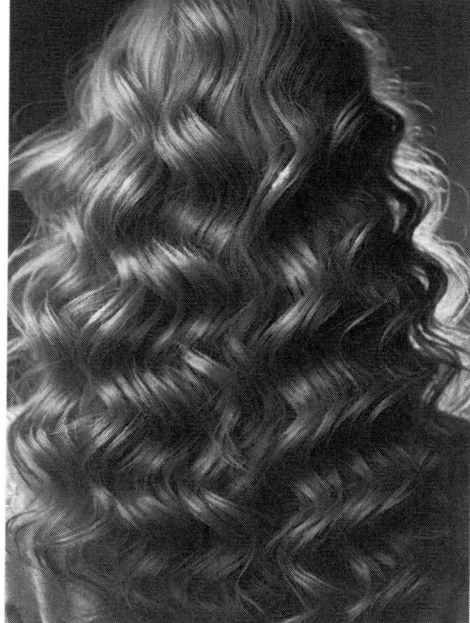

Step-by-Step Guide: Creating Romantic Curls

- Start with clean, dry hair.
- Apply a heat protectant spray to prevent damage.
- Use a curling iron or wand to take small sections of hair.

- Wrap each section around the barrel, hold for a few seconds, and release.
- Once all sections are curled, gently run your fingers through to loosen the curls.
- Spray with a light-hold hairspray to keep the curls in place without making them stiff.

Romantic curls are perfect for weddings or parties. They add a touch of glamour and are surprisingly easy to achieve. You'll look as if you stepped right out of a fairy tale.

5.3 Mastering The Art Of Blowouts

Alright, let's talk about blowouts. Ever wondered how to achieve that salon-quality blowout at home? It all starts with proper preparation. First, wash your hair with a volumizing shampoo. This helps to add body and lift from the get-go. Once you're out of the shower, gently towel dry your hair to remove excess water. Now, it's time for the magic potion: heat protectant. Apply it evenly throughout your damp hair. This step is crucial as it shields your strands from heat damage. Make sure to distribute the protectant well, from roots to tips. Now, section your hair into manageable parts. Use clips to keep each section separate. This makes the blow-drying process more efficient and ensures every part of your hair gets the attention it deserves.

Now, let's get to the blow-drying techniques that will give you that fabulous, bouncy blowout. Start by using a round brush. This tool is your best friend for creating volume and curl. Place the brush under a section of hair, starting at the roots, and aim the blow-dryer's nozzle down the hair shaft. This directional drying helps to smooth the cuticle and reduce frizz. Slowly move the brush and dryer down to the ends, following the brush with the airflow. Repeat this process for each section of hair until it's completely dry. For that final touch of salon magic, switch your dryer to the cool setting and give your hair a blast of cool air. This helps to set the style and add a bit of extra shine.

Volume and bounce are what make a blowout truly stand out. To achieve this, focus on lifting the roots. Use your round brush at the roots and pull upwards while blow-drying. This creates lift and gives your hair that coveted volume. If you want to go the extra mile, use rollers. After blow-drying each section, roll it up and secure it with a clip. Leave the rollers in until your hair cools down. This sets the shape and adds even more volume. When you take the rollers out, you'll be left with big, bouncy hair that looks like it's straight out of a magazine.

Maintaining your blowout is vital to keeping that fresh-from-the-salon look for as long as possible. Dry shampoo is a lifesaver here. It helps to absorb excess oil and keeps your hair looking fresh between washes. Simply spray it onto your roots, wait a few minutes, and then brush it out. For overnight maintenance, consider loosely tying your hair up in a bun or braids. This helps to preserve the shape and volume of your blowout while you sleep. A silk or satin pillowcase can also work wonders by reducing friction and preventing frizz. Lastly, avoid moisture at all costs. Use a shower cap when you're in the shower to keep your hair dry and protect your blowout from humidity.

With these tips and techniques, you'll be able to achieve and maintain a stunning blowout that looks like it was done by a professional. So go ahead, grab your tools, and get ready to flaunt that fabulous hair.

5.4 How To Style Hair For Volume And Texture

Let's be honest: who doesn't want hair that looks thick, full, and full of life? Adding volume and texture can completely transform your hairstyle, turning flat, lifeless locks into a glamorous mane. Volume gives the illusion of thicker hair, making every style look more robust and dynamic. Texture adds interest and movement, making your hair look effortlessly stylish. Imagine walking into a room and having your hair bounce with every step—it's a game changer.

One of the tried-and-true methods for adding volume is backcombing or teasing. This technique can give you that lift at the roots, making your hair look fuller. Start by sectioning off the top layer of your hair. Hold a section straight up and use a fine-tooth comb to comb downwards towards the scalp gently. This creates a cushion of hair that adds volume. Be careful not to go overboard, though; a few gentle strokes will do. Tease the roots in small sections for a more controlled, even lift. Once you've got that volume, smooth the top layer over to hide the teased sections. A light mist of hairspray will help hold everything in place without making it look stiff.

Texturizing products are your best friends when it comes to adding both volume and hold. Texturizing sprays and powders can give your hair that gritty, lived-in feel that makes it easier to style. Apply texturizing spray to dry hair, focusing on the roots for lift and the lengths for added texture. Work it in with your fingers to distribute the product evenly. Mousse is another fantastic option for adding volume. Apply a golf ball-sized amount of mousse to damp hair, working it through from roots to ends. Blow-dry using a round brush for maximum lift and bounce. The mousse helps to hold the volume and gives your hair a thicker appearance.

For those of you looking to take volume to the next level, Velcro rollers are a fantastic tool. After blow-drying a section of hair, wrap it around a Velcro roller and secure it at the scalp. Leave the rollers in while you finish your makeup or get dressed. The longer they stay in, the better the lift. Remove the rollers and gently brush through your hair for a bouncy, voluminous look. Blow-drying with a round brush is another excellent technique. Lift sections of hair at the roots with the brush and aim the blow dryer's nozzle down the hair shaft. This adds volume and smooths the hair, giving it a polished finish.

Layered cutting techniques can also add movement and texture to your hair. Layers remove some of the weight, allowing your hair to have more natural bounce and movement. Ask your stylist for layers that suit your hair type and desired look. Layers can be subtle for a natural effect or more pronounced for a dramatic change. They're especially effective for adding volume to fine hair, making it look fuller and more dynamic.

Adding volume and texture isn't just about making your hair look bigger; it's about creating styles that are full of life and movement. Whether you're teasing at the roots, using texturizing products, or incorporating layers, these techniques can help you achieve that voluminous, textured look that turns heads. So go ahead, play around with these tips, and watch your hair come to life.

5.5 Using Heat Tools: Best Practices And Safety Tips

Let's talk about heat tools, your trusty sidekicks for transforming your hair into whatever style you dream up. First, we've got flat irons. These bad boys are perfect for straightening your hair into sleek, shiny locks. But don't stop there—they can also create soft waves by twisting the iron as you glide it down your hair. Curling irons and wands are next on the list. Whether you're going for tight ringlets or loose beachy waves, these tools have you covered. Curling irons with clamps give you more control, while wands create more natural, free-flowing curls. Lastly, blow dryers are essential for volume and smoothness. They can be used with various attachments like diffusers for curly hair or concentrator nozzles for a sleek finish. Each tool has its unique perks, making them versatile for any style you want to achieve.

Safety first, folks! Heat tools can cause severe damage if not used properly. Always, and I mean always, use a heat protectant spray before applying any heat to your hair. This creates a barrier that helps prevent your hair from frying. Adjust the temperature based on your hair type. Fine or damaged hair requires a lower setting, while thicker hair can handle a bit more heat. Avoid excessive heat exposure by not going over the same section of hair multiple times. One good pass should do the trick. Trust me, your hair will thank you for it.

Now, let's get into some techniques for achieving those dreamy styles. To create beachy waves with a curling wand, start by sectioning your hair. Take a small section, wrap it around the wand (away from your face), and hold for a few seconds. Release and let the curl cool for a bit before running your fingers through it for a relaxed look. To straighten your hair while maintaining volume, use a flat iron at the roots and pull upwards before gliding it down. This lifts the roots and adds a bit of oomph. If you're aiming for a salon-quality blowout, use a round brush to lift sections of hair at the roots while directing the blow dryer's nozzle down the shaft. This not only smooths the hair but also adds incredible volume and shine.

Taking care of your heat tools is just as important as using them correctly. Clean the plates of your flat iron regularly to remove any product buildup. A damp cloth usually does the trick. Always check the cords and plugs for any signs of wear and tear. Safety first, remember? Store your tools properly to avoid damage. A heat-resistant mat or pouch is excellent for this. It keeps the tools safe and ensures they last longer.

Heat tools can be your best friend when it comes to styling your hair, but you've got to treat them right. Using them safely and effectively can make a world of difference in achieving those fabulous looks while keeping your hair healthy. So, go ahead, pick up that flat iron or curling wand, and get ready to style away, knowing you've got the skills and knowledge to do it right.

5.6 Experimenting With Hair Accessories: Clips,

Bands, And More

Alright, let's talk about hair accessories. These little gems can transform even the most straightforward hairstyle into a head-turner. First up, we have decorative clips and pins. Think of them as jewelry for your hair. They come in all shapes, sizes, and designs— from sparkly rhinestones to elegant pearls. These are perfect for adding a touch of glam to any look. Then, there are headbands and bandanas. These are not just for keeping your hair out of your face; they're fashion statements. Whether you're rocking a sporty look or channeling your inner boho chic, there's a headband or bandana for every occasion. Lastly, hair scarves and wraps are the ultimate versatile accessory. You can tie them around your head like a headband, weave them into a braid, or wrap them around a bun for that effortlessly cool vibe.

Now, let's get into how to incorporate these accessories into your hairstyles. Imagine you've just finished a simple braid. Nice, but a bit plain, right? Add a decorative clip or pin near the base, and suddenly, it's elegant enough for a night out. Headbands are another game-changer. They're perfect for those days when your hair won't cooperate. Slip one on, and voilà, instant style and function. They're also great for keeping your hair off your face during workouts or study sessions. For a more relaxed, boho look, try wrapping a scarf around a messy bun. It adds a pop of color and makes the bun look intentional rather than a last-minute fix.

Ready to take it up a notch? Let's talk about advanced accessory techniques. Want to create a faux bob without the commitment of a haircut? Use a headband. Place it over your head, then tuck your hair up and under the band to create the illusion of shorter hair. It's a fun way to switch things up without the scissors. For a decorative updo, use multiple pins. Start with a simple twist or bun, then add several decorative pins in a pattern. It turns a basic style into a work of art. You can even mix and match different pins for a unique look.

Choosing the right accessories can make or break your hairstyle. Match your accessories to your outfit and the occasion.

A sparkly clip might be perfect for a party but out of place at a casual hangout. Consider the colors and patterns too. Accessories that complement your hair color can make the style pop. For instance, gold looks stunning against dark hair, while silver shines on lighter locks. Also, think about the weight and size of the accessories. Heavy clips can be uncomfortable and might not stay in place, especially if you have fine hair. Opt for lighter, more secure options for all-day comfort.

Experimenting with hair accessories is a fun and easy way to elevate your hairstyles. Whether you're adding a clip to a braid, slipping on a headband, or wrapping a scarf around a bun, these little additions can make a significant impact. So, grab an accessory and get creative next time you're feeling a bit blah about your hair. You might be surprised at how much it can transform your look.

5.7 Mastering Hair Extensions And Wigs

Let's talk about hair extensions and wigs—your secret weapons for instant length, volume, and versatility. If you've ever dreamed of long, luscious locks or just wanted to switch up your style without the commitment, extensions and wigs are your go-to. First up, let's dive into the different types of hair extensions. Clip-in extensions are the easiest and most temporary option. They're perfect for adding length and volume in a snap, and can be removed just as quickly. Simply snap them in and out whenever you feel like changing up your look. They're great for special occasions or when you want to add a bit of drama to your everyday style.

Next, we have tape-in extensions, which offer a more semi-permanent solution. These extensions use a special adhesive to bond to your natural hair and can last several weeks. They lie flat against your scalp, making them less noticeable and more comfortable than some other types. They're ideal if you want a longer-lasting style but aren't quite ready for the commitment of sew-in extensions. Speaking of which, sew-in extensions are the most long-lasting option. They're literally sewn into your natural hair, providing a secure and durable way to add length and volume. These are perfect for those who want a more permanent change and are okay with a bit of extra maintenance.

Now, let's weigh the pros and cons. Clip-in extensions are super convenient and versatile. You can put them in and take them out whenever you like, making them perfect for those who frequently switch up their style. However, they can be tricky to blend with your natural hair if not done correctly. Tape-in extensions offer a more seamless look and are less likely to cause damage to your natural hair. On the downside, the adhesive can sometimes cause irritation, and you'll need to be cautious with heat styling. Sew-in extensions provide the most natural and long-lasting results but come with their own set of challenges. They can be heavy and put a strain on your natural hair, requiring regular maintenance and care.

Let's not forget about wigs. These are fantastic for completely transforming your look without any long-term commitment. Wigs come in all styles, lengths, and colors, allowing you to experiment with different looks. They're perfect for those who want to try out a new style without making a permanent change. Plus, they're a lifesaver on bad hair days. However, finding the right fit and ensuring it looks natural can be a challenge. High-quality wigs can also be pricey, but they're worth the investment if you plan to wear them often.

So, whether you're looking to add some temporary length for a special occasion or want a more permanent change, hair extensions and wigs have got you covered. They offer endless possibilities for creativity and self-expression, allowing you to play around with different looks and find what suits you best. With a bit of practice and care, you'll be able to seamlessly integrate them into your routine and rock any style with confidence.

Wrapping Up Chapter 5

So, there you have it—advanced styling techniques that will make you feel like a hair pro. From mastering braids to adding volume and experimenting with extensions, these skills open up a world of possibilities. Next up, we'll explore how to keep your hair healthy and robust, ensuring it always looks its best. Stay tuned!

CHAPTER 6: PROTECTIVE STYLES AND MAINTENANCE

Imagine this: you've just spent an hour detangling, moisturizing, and styling your hair to perfection, only to step outside and have it ruined by humidity or wind in seconds. We've all been there, right? But what if I told you there's a way to keep your hair looking fabulous with minimal effort? Enter the world of protective styles. These are your hair's best friends, especially when you want to give it a break from daily styling and manipulation.

6.1 Understanding Protective Styles

So, what exactly are protective styles? Simply put, these are hairstyles that tuck away the ends of your hair, minimizing manipulation and shielding it from environmental damage. Picture protective styles as a cozy blanket for your hair, keeping it safe and snug. They're essential for maintaining healthy hair because they reduce breakage and allow your hair to rest and grow. When you're constantly styling and combing your hair, you're putting stress on it, which can lead to breakage. Protective styles help to minimize this daily wear and tear.

One of the biggest perks of protective styles is that they shield your hair from environmental damage. Think about it: sun, wind, and pollution can wreak havoc on your hair, making it dry and brittle. By tucking your hair away in a protective style, you're giving it a barrier against these harsh elements. Plus, protective styles promote hair growth by allowing your hair to rest. When your hair isn't being constantly manipulated, it has a chance to grow stronger and longer.

There are several types of protective styles to choose from, each with its own unique benefits. Braids are a popular choice, and they come in many forms, from box braids to cornrows. Box braids are individual plaits that can last for weeks, while cornrows are braids that lie flat against your scalp. Both styles are great for keeping your hair protected and low-maintenance. Twists are another excellent option. Two-strand twists involve twisting two sections of hair together.

In contrast, Senegalese twists use hair extensions to create a thicker, fuller look. Updos like buns and chignons are also fantastic for keeping your hair tucked away and protected. And let's not forget about wigs and weaves. These full-coverage options allow you to switch up your look while keeping your natural hair safe and sound underneath.

The benefits of incorporating protective styles into your hair care routine are endless. For starters, they help with moisture retention. When your hair is tucked away, it's less likely to lose moisture, keeping it hydrated and healthy. Protective styles are also time-savers. Once your hair is styled, you don't have to worry about daily styling, which means more time for you to focus on other things. And let's talk about versatility. With protective styles, you can switch up your look without causing damage to your natural hair. Want long, flowing locks one day and a chic bob the next? Protective styles make it possible.

Choosing the right protective style depends on your hair type and texture. If you have fine hair, you'll want to opt for lightweight styles that won't weigh your hair down or cause breakage. Think loose twists or a simple updo. For those with thick hair, styles that manage volume are critical. Box braids or chunky twists can help keep your hair under control while still looking fabulous. Coily hair benefits from styles that reduce shrinkage and keep your curls stretched out. Two-strand twists or cornrows are excellent options for protecting and stretching your hair.

Protective styles are a game-changer for anyone looking to maintain healthy hair with minimal effort. They reduce breakage, shield your hair from environmental damage, and promote growth by allowing it to rest. Plus, they're versatile and time-saving, making them perfect for busy lifestyles. Whether you choose braids, twists, updos, or wigs, there's a protective style that's perfect for you. So give your hair the break it deserves and enjoy the benefits of protective styling.

6.2 How To Do Box Braids

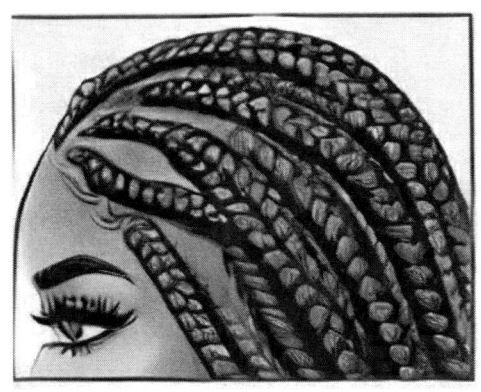

I am not experienced in any way with Box Braids, and I feel that pictures do not give you the idea and ability for you to grasp how to properly box braid. With that being said here is some articles and videos that I think will help and guide you:

- **Learn How to Create, Style, and Care for Your Own Box Braids https://www.wikihow.com/Do-Box-Braids**
- **DIY BOX BRAIDS: 3 Easy Simple techniques for Beginner Braiders https://**

www.curlynikki.com/2023/09/box-braids-3-simple-techniques.html

This creator has her video linked at the bottom of her article!

- ****VERY DETAILED** How To Start A Box Braid TUTORIAL |·3 Different Methods |·BraidsbyTyTi** https://www.youtube.com/watch?v=vNFTB08b1tw
This creator has a bunch of comments that say that this video is a great resource for beginners!

Alright, you're ready to take the plunge into the fabulous world of box braids. First things first, preparation is key. Think of it as prepping for a big event—your hair needs to be clean, detangled, and moisturized. Start by washing your hair with a gentle shampoo to remove any buildup. Follow up with a good conditioner to make detangling easier. Once you're out of the shower, gently detangle your hair using a wide-tooth comb, starting from the ends and working your way up to the roots. Trust me, your fingers and scalp will thank you later for this step.

Next, you'll want to section your hair into uniform parts. This is where your rat-tail comb becomes your best friend. Create sections that are about the size of the braids you want. Smaller sections mean more braids and potentially more time, while larger sections mean fewer braids and a quicker process. Clip or tie each section to keep them separated. This makes the braiding process smoother and helps ensure that your braids are neat and even. Once your hair is sectioned, apply a leave-in conditioner to keep it moisturized and manageable throughout the braiding process. A little bit of extra love here will go a long way in keeping your hair healthy under the braids.

Now, let's get into the nitty-gritty of creating those box braids.

Start by taking a small section of hair from one of your pre-made parts. Use your rat-tail comb to create a clean, straight line. If you're adding extensions, this is the time to blend them with your natural hair. Fold the extension so that it's even on both sides. Place it at the root of your hair section and begin braiding, incorporating your natural hair with the extension. Keep the tension even but not too tight—you don't want to end up with a headache or damage your hair. As you braid down, make sure the braid stays tight and uniform. Once you reach the end, you have a few options for securing it. You can burn the ends with a lighter, dip them in hot water, or use rubber bands. Each method has its own pros and cons, so choose the one that works best for you.

Maintaining your box braids is just as important as the installation. Start with scalp care. Apply oils like jojoba or coconut oil to keep your scalp moisturized and itch-free. Using a nozzle bottle can help you get the oil right where it's needed without making a mess. When it comes to washing your braids, be gentle. Use a diluted shampoo mixture and focus on your scalp, letting the suds run down the braids. Rinse thoroughly and follow up with a light conditioner. Preventing frizz is also crucial to keeping your braids looking fresh. A mousse or gel can help smooth flyaways and give your braids a sleek finish.

Eventually, the time will come to remove your box braids. It's crucial to do this carefully to avoid damaging your hair. Start by cutting the ends of the braids, making sure not to cut your natural hair. Then, unravel the braids gently. Use a detangling spray or conditioner to make the process easier. Once all the braids are out, give your hair a thorough wash and deep conditioning treatment. Your hair has been tucked away for a while, so it deserves some extra TLC.

Box braids are a fantastic protective style that can be both stylish and practical. With the proper preparation, technique, and maintenance, you'll be rocking those braids like a pro.

6.3 Maintaining And Caring For Twists

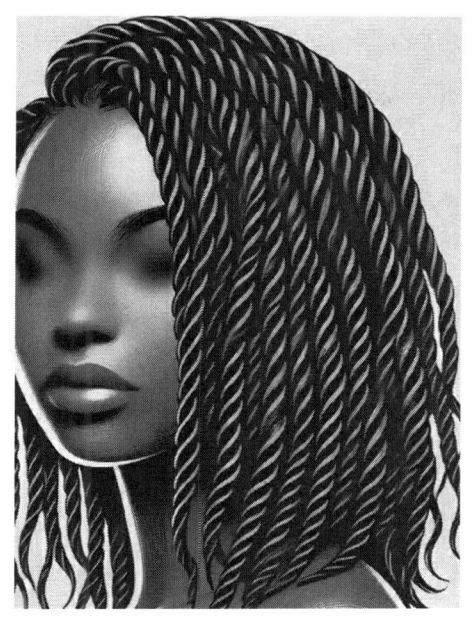

As I said with the box braids, I am not experienced in any way with Twists, and I feel that pictures do not give you the idea and ability for you to grasp how to properly create twists. With that being said here is some articles and videos that I think will help and guide you:

- **Twisting Your Own Hair at Home: A Step-By-Step Guide** https://www.wikihow.com/Twist-Hair
- **How to twist your own hair at home** https://www.youtube.com/watch?&v=m91okpJkDWU
- **Twist and Turn Two Strand Twists- Natural Hair Style** https://www.curlynikki.com/2023/11/twist-and-turn-

two-strand-twists.html

Twists are like the Swiss Army knife of protective styles—versatile, effective, and suitable for just about any occasion. There are different types of twists, each with its own benefits. Two-strand twists are your go-to for simplicity and effectiveness. They involve dividing a section of hair into two parts and twisting them around each other. This style is perfect if you want something quick and easy that still looks polished. Marley twists to take it up a notch by incorporating Marley hair extensions, giving your hair added length and volume. These twists are great if you're looking for a fuller look without the commitment of permanent extensions. Then we have Havana twists, which are larger and more voluminous. These twists use thicker extensions and give you that big, bold look that's perfect for making a statement.

Creating twists is a straightforward process, but it does require some prep work. Start by sectioning your hair to ensure uniformity. This makes the twisting process smoother and ensures that each twist is consistent. Use a rat-tail comb to create clean parts, and clip away sections you're not working on to keep things organized. When you're ready to twist, take a small section of hair and divide it into two parts. Maintain even tension as you twist the two strands around each other. This helps keep the twists neat and prevents them from unraveling. Secure the ends with rubber bands or small clips to keep them in place. If you're using extensions, blend them with your natural hair as you twist for a seamless look.

Maintaining twists daily is all about keeping them moisturized and frizz-free. Use a spray bottle filled with a mixture of water and conditioner to keep your twists hydrated. Give your hair a light spritz each morning to maintain moisture levels. For scalp care, apply light oils like jojoba or argan oil. These oils help keep your scalp moisturized without making your hair greasy. Just a few drops massaged into your scalp can make a big difference. Wrap your hair in a satin scarf or bonnet before bed to prevent frizz. Satin reduces friction, helping to keep your twists smooth and intact while you sleep.

Refreshing your twists is crucial for prolonging their lifespan and keeping them looking fresh. If your twists start to look a little tired, give them a quick spritz with your water and conditioner mixture. This helps to reactivate any product already in your hair and gives your twists a little boost. For more stubborn frizz, apply a small amount of styling gel or mousse to smooth things down. You can also re-twist any sections that have started to unravel. Simply take the section, reapply some moisture, and twist it back up. This quick touch-up can make a world of difference in the overall appearance of your twists.

Twists are a fantastic protective style that offers both versatility and ease of maintenance. Whether you're rocking two-strand twists, Marley twists, or Havana twists, consistent care is the key to keeping them looking great. By keeping your twists moisturized, maintaining your scalp, and taking steps to prevent frizz, you can enjoy a stylish and low-maintenance look that lasts. So go ahead, give twists a try, and see just how easy and effective this protective style can be.

6.4 The Benefits Of Wearing Wigs

Let's talk wigs—a total game-changer for anyone looking to switch up their look without making a long-term commitment. Wigs offer a world of possibilities, from protecting your natural hair to giving you the freedom to experiment with different styles. If you've ever wanted to go from a pixie cut to waist-length waves overnight, wigs are your best friend. They're versatile, stylish, and a lifesaver on bad hair days.

There are several types of wigs, each with its own unique benefits. Lace-front wigs are a popular choice because they offer a natural-looking hairline. The lace front blends seamlessly with your skin, making it look like the hair is growing right out of your scalp. These wigs are great if you want to pull your hair back into a ponytail or an updo without revealing that you're wearing a wig. Full lace wigs take it a step further by offering versatility in styling. With a full lace wig, you can part your hair any way you like and even wear it in braids or high ponytails. It's like having a blank canvas to create any look you desire.

When it comes to choosing between synthetic and human hair wigs, there are pros and cons for both. Synthetic wigs are generally more affordable and come pre-styled, so they're ready to wear immediately. They also hold their style well, even after washing. However, they can't be heat-styled, so you're stuck with the style it comes in. On the other hand, human hair wigs offer a natural look and feel. You can style them just like your natural hair with heat tools, and they tend to last longer with proper care. The downside? They're more expensive and require more maintenance.

Choosing the right wig involves a few key considerations. First, match the wig's texture to your natural hair. This helps blend the wig with your hairline and makes it look more realistic. If your natural hair is curly, opt for a curly wig. If it's straight, go for straight styles. Next, consider the wig cap construction. You want something comfortable and breathable, especially if you intend to wear the wig for extended periods. Look for wigs with adjustable straps and breathable materials to ensure a snug but comfortable fit. Color selection is also crucial. Choose a color that complements your skin tone. If you're unsure, stick with shades close to your natural hair color. Once you're more comfortable, you can experiment with bolder colors.

Applying and securing a wig properly can make all the difference in achieving a seamless look. Start with a wig cap to create a smooth base. This helps keep your natural hair flat and secure under the wig. Next, use adhesives or clips to secure the wig in place. Wig adhesives, such as glue or tape, offer a reliable grip to ensure your wig stays securely in place. While clips are quick and easy to use. Once the wig is on, blend it with your natural hair. Use a bit of concealer or foundation on the lace front to match your skin tone, and style the baby hairs to create a natural hairline.

Maintaining your wig is essential for ensuring its longevity. For synthetic wigs, use products specifically designed for synthetic hair. Gently detangle the wig with a wide-tooth comb and wash it with a mild shampoo. Let it air dry on a wig stand to maintain its shape. Human hair wigs require a bit more care. Use sulfate-free shampoos and conditioners to keep the hair moisturized. Detangle gently and avoid excessive heat styling to prevent damage. Store your wig on a wig stand or in a silk bag to keep it in top condition.

Wearing wigs opens up a world of styling possibilities while protecting your natural hair. Whether you choose lace front, full lace, synthetic, or human hair wigs, the key is to find what works best for you and your lifestyle. With the right wig, you can change your look instantly and enjoy the freedom of experimenting with different styles without the commitment. So go ahead, have fun with it, and let your creativity shine through.

6.5 Protective Styles For Sports And Exercise

When it comes to hitting the gym, running track, or even practicing yoga, the last thing you want is hair getting in your way. Choosing practical styles for physical activity is vital to keeping your hair protected while you break a sweat. Braids are a fantastic option. Cornrows lie flat against your scalp, making them perfect for high-intensity workouts. Boxer or double French braids offer a secure and stylish way to keep your hair tamed. If you're more into buns, high and low buns work wonders. They keep your hair up and out of your face, which is especially handy for activities like running or cycling. Twists are another great choice. Flat twists or twisted updos keep your hair neatly secured, reducing the risk of tangling or breakage.

Before you even start your workout, a good pre-exercise hair care routine sets the stage for keeping your hair in top shape. Moisturizing is crucial. Applying a leave-in conditioner can help keep your hair hydrated, even as you sweat. It acts as a barrier, preventing sweat from drying out your hair. Securing your hair with non-damaging hair ties is another must. Regular elastics can cause breakage, so opt for ones made from softer materials like fabric-covered bands. To top it all off, wearing a sweat-wicking headband can absorb moisture and keep your hairline dry. It's like giving your hair a little spa treatment before you start exercising.

Post-exercise hair care is just as crucial as pre-exercise prep. Sweat can make your scalp feel gross and itchy, so it's essential to remove it properly. Start by using a damp cloth to gently wipe away sweat from your scalp and hairline. This helps to remove excess salt and prevent buildup. Refreshing your scalp with a scalp spray can also work wonders. Look for sprays that contain ingredients like tea tree oil or peppermint; they're great for soothing and cooling your scalp. Finally, re-moisturize your hair with light oils or serums. Just a few drops can help restore hydration and keep your hair looking fresh and healthy.

Maintaining your protective styles during workouts is all about making small adjustments to keep everything in place. If you're rocking braids, make sure to secure the ends with a little extra care. Using additional elastics or even small clips can prevent them from unraveling. For buns, a few strategically placed bobby pins can keep everything locked down, even during high-impact activities. Twists can benefit from a bit of extra gel or mousse applied before your workout to keep them neat and frizz-free. And please remember that headband—it's your best friend when it comes to keeping your edges intact and absorbing sweat.

Selecting the right protective styles and maintaining them during physical activities doesn't have to be a hassle. With a bit of prep and the proper techniques, you can keep your hair looking fabulous and healthy, no matter how intense your workout gets. Whether you're into braids, buns, or twists, there's a protective style out there that's perfect for your active lifestyle. So go ahead, break a sweat, and let your hair stay as strong and resilient as you are.

6.6 Nighttime Routines For Hair Protection

Do you know how you spend all that time making your hair look flawless, only to wake up looking like you were wrestling with a tornado? Nighttime protection is crucial for keeping your hair healthy and looking good. When you sleep, friction between your hair and pillow can cause breakage. Imagine your hair rubbing against a rough surface for hours—yikes! It's like using sandpaper on your strands. Protecting your hair at night helps prevent this damage. Plus, it retains moisture, which is essential for avoiding that dry, brittle feeling. No one wants to wake up with hair as dry as a desert.

Enter satin and silk accessories. These are game-changers for nighttime hair care. Satin bonnets, for example, keep your hair secure while you sleep. They're like cozy little sleeping bags for your locks. By reducing friction, satin bonnets help prevent breakage and keep your hair smooth. Silk pillowcases are another fantastic option. Unlike cotton, silk reduces friction and helps your hair retain moisture. So even if you toss and turn, your hair stays protected. Then there are satin scarves, which you can wrap around your hair to keep it in place. They're perfect for those who don't like the feel of a bonnet but still want the benefits of reduced friction.

When it comes to nighttime styling techniques, you've got a few options to keep your hair protected. If you have curly or coily hair, the pineappling method is a lifesaver. It involves gathering your hair into a high, loose ponytail on top of your head. This keeps your curls intact and prevents them from getting squished while you sleep. Loose braids are another great option. Braiding your hair loosely helps prevent tangles and keeps your hair organized. It's like giving your hair a little bedtime routine of its own. Twisting your hair is another method that works wonders for maintaining definition. Just twist sections of your hair before bed, and you'll wake up with defined curls or waves.

Refreshing your hair in the morning doesn't have to be a hassle. Start with a spray bottle filled with water or a water-conditioner mix. Give your hair a light spritz to reactivate any product and bring your curls back to life. It's like hitting the refresh button on your hair. Applying light oils can also add shine and reduce frizz. Just a few drops of Argan or Jojoba oil can make a big difference. Finally, quick styles like buns or ponytails are your best friends for those mornings when you're in a rush. They're easy to do and keep your hair looking polished without much effort.

So, protecting your hair at night is a must if you want to keep it healthy and looking its best. From satin and silk accessories to simple nighttime styles, there are plenty of ways to give your hair the love it needs while you catch some Z's. And with a few quick tips for refreshing your hair in the morning, you'll be ready to take on the day with fabulous locks.

Wrapping Up Chapter 6

Protective styles and nighttime routines are your secret weapons for maintaining healthy, beautiful hair. From choosing the right style for daily wear to ensuring your hair stays protected during sleep, these techniques make a world of difference. Next, we'll explore how to address common hair problems, offering solutions that keep your hair looking its best.

CHAPTER 7: ADDRESSING COMMON HAIR PROBLEMS

Ever had one of those days when your hair looks like you've just stuck your finger in an electrical socket? Yep, we're talking frizz. It's the nemesis of smooth, sleek hair and a common struggle for many. Let's dive into what causes this hair-raising issue and how to tame it once and for all.

7.1 Frizz Control: Techniques And Products That Work

So, what's the deal with frizz? It all starts with humidity and moisture in the air. When the air is humid, your hair absorbs the extra moisture, causing the cuticle to swell and lift. This makes your hair look like it's trying to escape from your head. Lack of proper hydration is another biggie. If your hair is dry, it'll suck up any moisture it can find, including that pesky humidity. And let's not forget over-styling and heat damage. Using hot tools too often can strip your hair of its natural oils, leaving it dry and frizz-prone. Basically, it's like your hair is throwing a frizz party, and everyone's invited.

Now, let's talk about the heavy hitters in the anti-frizz product lineup. Anti-frizz serums and leave-in conditioners are like magic potions for your hair. They coat your strands, locking in moisture and keeping the frizz at bay. Products like **TRESemme Keratin**

Smooth Shine Serum are top-notch for this. Smoothing creams and oils, like **BioSilk Silk Therapy with Natural Coconut Oil Leave-In Treatment**, are also fantastic. They add a layer of protection and help smooth down the cuticle. And if you're battling humidity, humidity-resistant sprays are your new best friend. They create a barrier against the moisture in the air, keeping your hair sleek and smooth.

When it comes to taming frizz, the technique is everything. First off, ditch that regular towel and switch to a microfiber towel to dry your hair. Regular towels can rough up the cuticle, making frizz worse. Microfiber towels are gentler and help reduce friction. After washing, apply your anti-frizz products to damp hair. This helps lock in moisture and sets the stage for smooth styling. And for the love of all things hair, avoid excessive brushing. Brushing can break up your hair's natural wave pattern, leading to—you guessed it—frizz. Use a wide-tooth comb instead, and only when your hair is wet.

Feeling DIY? There are plenty of natural remedies you can whip up at home to combat frizz. Aloe vera gel is a superstar when it comes to hydration. Apply a small amount to damp hair to seal in moisture and add shine. Coconut oil treatments are another great option. Warm up a bit of coconut oil and apply it to your hair, focusing on the ends. Leave it on for about 30 minutes, then rinse. Your hair will feel like silk. Apple cider vinegar rinses can also help. Mix one part apple cider vinegar with two parts water and rinse your hair with it after shampooing. It helps smooth the cuticle and adds a lovely shine.

Frizz doesn't have to be a permanent guest in your hair. With the right products, techniques, and a little bit of DIY magic, you can keep those unruly strands in check and enjoy smooth, sleek hair every day.

7.2 Preventing And Repairing Hair Breakage

Ever feel like your hair is more fragile than your grandma's fine china? Hair breakage can be a real pain, but knowing what causes it can help you avoid those pesky split ends and broken strands. One primary culprit is over-processing with chemicals. Think about all those times you've bleached, dyed, or chemically straightened your hair. Each of those processes weakens your hair structure, making it more prone to breakage. Excessive heat styling is another enemy. Using high-temperature tools like flat irons and curling wands without proper protection can fry your hair, turning it into a brittle mess. And let's not forget about physical damage from tight hairstyles. Constantly pulling your hair into tight ponytails or braids can put a lot of stress on your strands, leading to breakage over time.

But don't worry, you're not doomed to a life of shattered strands. There are plenty of products designed to strengthen your hair and prevent breakage. Protein treatments are fantastic for this. They work by filling in the gaps in your hair shaft, making it stronger and more resilient. Products like Olaplex No. 3 Hair Perfector are great for this. Bond-building products are another excellent option. They help to repair and strengthen the internal structure of your hair, giving it more elasticity and reducing breakage. Strengthening shampoos and conditioners, like those from the Living Proof Restore line, can also make a big difference. They fortify your hair with each wash, helping to keep it strong and healthy.

Handling your hair properly can also go a long way in preventing breakage. First off, switch to a wide-tooth comb or a detangling brush. These tools are gentler on your hair and help to reduce breakage when you're detangling. Avoid tight hairstyles and hair ties that can put stress on your strands. Instead, opt for looser styles and use fabric-covered hair ties. And be extra careful when your hair is wet. Wet hair is more fragile and prone to breakage, so handle it with care. Use a microfiber towel to gently blot your hair dry and avoid rubbing it vigorously.

If your hair is already showing signs of breakage, don't panic. There are plenty of treatments that can help repair the damage. Reparative hair masks are a great place to start. They provide deep conditioning and help to strengthen your hair from the inside out. Look for masks that contain ingredients like keratin or biotin. Leave-in conditioners and serums are also fantastic for adding moisture and reducing breakage. Apply them to damp hair to lock in hydration and protect your strands. Finally, consider using a bond-building treatment like Olaplex No. 0 and No. 3. These products work together to repair the internal structure of your hair, making it stronger and less prone to breakage.

Understanding what leads to hair breakage and taking steps to prevent it can save you a lot of heartache—and hair ache. By using the right products and handling your hair with care, you can keep your locks strong and healthy. So go ahead, give your hair the love it deserves, and say goodbye to breakage for good.

7.3 Preventing And Treating Split Ends

Ever noticed those annoying little white tips at the ends of your hair? Yep, those are split ends, and they're the bane of anyone trying to grow out their locks. Split ends happen when the protective outer layer of your hair cuticle wears away due to various forms of damage. Heat damage is a primary culprit here. Frequent use of styling tools like flat irons, curling wands, and even blow dryers can cause the hair shaft to weaken and split. Another big offender is mechanical damage. Aggressive brushing, especially when your hair is wet, can cause your strands to fray and split. It's like trying to untangle a necklace by yanking at it—you're bound to break something.

So, how do you keep split ends at bay? Regular trims are your first line of defense. Aim to trim your hair every 6–8 weeks. This might sound counterintuitive if you're trying to grow your hair out, but cutting off the damaged ends actually helps your hair look healthier and less prone to breaking further. Using heat protectants is another crucial step. Before you go to town with any hot tools, spritz your hair with a heat protectant spray. This creates a barrier that helps minimize heat damage. And, if you can, give your hair a break from the heat whenever possible. Embrace your natural texture or try heatless styling methods.

But what if you already have split ends? While the only surefire way to get rid of them is to cut them off, there are treatments that can help manage and temporarily fix them. Split-end menders are products designed to seal the broken ends together, making them less noticeable. They're not a permanent fix, but they can hold things together until your next trim. Deep conditioning treatments are also fantastic for keeping your hair hydrated and less prone to splitting. Aim to deep condition at least once a week. Protein treatments can also help strengthen your hair, making it more resilient to damage. These treatments fill in the gaps in your hair shaft, fortifying it from the inside out.

Feeling crafty? DIY remedies can work wonders for split ends. An egg yolk and olive oil mask is a fantastic option. Mix one egg yolk with two tablespoons of olive oil, apply it to your hair, and let it sit for about 20 minutes before rinsing. The protein in the egg helps strengthen your hair, while the olive oil adds much-needed moisture. Coconut oil is another great treatment. Warm up a bit of coconut oil and apply it to your hair, focusing on the ends. Leave it on for about 30 minutes before washing it out. Your hair will feel softer and more manageable. Shea butter is also a fantastic natural remedy. Melt a small amount between your fingers and apply it to the ends of your hair. It's rich in vitamins and fatty acids that help nourish and protect your hair.

Split ends might be a common problem, but they're not unbeatable. By understanding what causes them and taking proactive steps to prevent and treat them, you can keep your hair looking healthy and vibrant. Regular trims, heat protectants, and deep conditioning are your best friends in this battle. And for those times when you need a little extra help, don't underestimate the power of a good DIY treatment. So go ahead, pamper those ends, and keep your hair looking its best.

7.4 Remedies For Dry And Itchy Scalp

Ever scratch your head and feel like you might strike oil? A dry and itchy scalp can be a real nuisance, turning you into a human snow globe with flakes everywhere. Several factors can contribute to this discomfort. Environmental conditions like cold weather can strip your scalp of its natural moisture, leaving it dry and itchy. Overusing harsh hair products, like those loaded with sulfates, can also wreak havoc, stripping your scalp of its natural oils and causing irritation. And let's not forget skin conditions like eczema or psoriasis, which can make your scalp feel like it's on fire.

To soothe your scalp, you need products designed to hydrate and calm it down. Scalp oils and serums are fantastic for this. Products like Gisou Honey-Infused Scalp Treatment Serum are packed with moisturizing ingredients like honey and glycerin, which help to soothe and hydrate your scalp. Hydrating shampoos and conditioners, such as those from the TSD Hair Flower Extract line, can also make a big difference. These products are formulated to add moisture and reduce dryness. Leave-in treatments are another great option. They provide ongoing hydration and protection, keeping your scalp comfortable throughout the day.

If you're into DIY remedies, there are plenty of natural treatments you can try at home. A coconut oil and tea tree oil massage is a great place to start. Coconut oil is deeply hydrating, while tea tree oil has antifungal properties that can help soothe an itchy scalp. Mix a few drops of tea tree oil with a tablespoon of coconut oil, massage it into your scalp, and let it sit for about 30 minutes before rinsing. Another option is aloe vera gel. It's incredibly soothing and can help to calm any irritation. Apply it directly to your scalp and let it sit for 20 minutes before rinsing. If you're feeling adventurous, try an oatmeal and honey scalp mask. Mix equal parts of oatmeal and honey, apply to your scalp, and leave it on for 20 minutes. It's like a spa day for your scalp.

Maintaining a healthy scalp requires a bit of TLC. Regular gentle exfoliation can help remove any buildup of dead skin cells and promote a healthier scalp. Look for products with gentle exfoliants like salicylic acid. Avoid washing your hair with hot water, as it can strip your scalp of its natural oils. Stick to lukewarm or cool water instead. If you live in a particularly dry climate, using a humidifier can help add moisture to the air, keeping your scalp from drying out. These simple practices can make a big difference in keeping your scalp healthy and itch-free.

A healthy scalp is the foundation for beautiful hair. By understanding the causes of dryness and itchiness and taking proactive steps to address them, you can keep your scalp comfortable and your hair looking its best. So, pamper your scalp with some much-needed moisture and enjoy the benefits of healthy, happy hair.

7.5 Managing Oily Hair And Scalp

Ever feel like your hair has its own oil slick happening? Oily hair and scalp can be a real drag, and the struggle is real for many of us. The main culprit behind all that grease is overactive sebaceous glands. These little guys work overtime, producing more oil than your scalp needs. Hormonal changes, like those during puberty or monthly cycles, can also throw your oil production into overdrive. Then there's product buildup. Using too many products or not rinsing them out properly can leave a residue that makes your hair look greasy even when it's clean. It's like your hair is holding on to every drop of product for dear life.

To keep that oil in check, you need the right products. Clarifying shampoos are a lifesaver. They're designed to remove product buildup and excess oil, leaving your scalp feeling fresh and clean. A good one to try is Neutrogena Anti-Residue Shampoo. For conditioning, go for something lightweight. Heavy conditioners can weigh your hair down and make it greasy faster. Dry shampoos are also your best friend. They soak up excess oil and give your hair a clean, fresh look without having to wash it. Batiste Dry Shampoo is a popular choice that works wonders.

When washing your oily hair, technique matters. Use lukewarm water instead of hot. Hot water can stimulate your sebaceous glands to produce even more oil. Focus on your scalp when shampooing. Apply the shampoo to your roots and massage gently with your fingertips, then let the suds work their way down to the ends. This helps to remove oil and buildup from your scalp where it's needed most. When it's time to condition, only apply it to the ends of your hair. Your roots don't need the extra moisture, and it'll just make your hair greasy faster.

Managing oily hair between washes can be tricky, but it's doable with a few handy tips. Blotting papers aren't just for your face. You can use them on your scalp to absorb excess oil throughout the day. It's a quick fix when you're on the go and need to freshen up. Keeping your hairbrushes clean is also crucial. Dirty brushes can transfer oil and product buildup back onto your hair, making it greasy again. Give them a good wash regularly to keep them clean. Avoid heavy styling products that can weigh your hair down and add to the oiliness. Opt for lighter options that won't contribute to the grease fest.

Managing oily hair and scalp might seem like a never-ending battle, but with the right products and techniques, you can keep the oil at bay and enjoy fresh, clean hair every day.

7.6 How To Deal With Hair Loss And Thinning

Hair loss and thinning can feel like a nightmare, especially when you're brushing your hair and end up with a handful of strands. It's not just a bad hair day; it's a bad hair month. Several factors contribute to this issue. Genetic predispositions play a significant role. If your family has a history of hair loss, chances are you might experience it too. Hormonal imbalances, such as those caused by thyroid issues or hormonal changes during puberty and menopause, can also mess with your hair's growth cycle. Nutritional deficiencies are another common culprit. A lack of essential vitamins and minerals, like iron or vitamin D, can weaken your hair and lead to thinning. And let's not forget stress and medical conditions. High-stress levels and conditions like alopecia can lead to significant hair loss.

When it comes to tackling hair loss, there are several products designed to promote growth and reduce thinning. **Minoxidil** treatments are a popular choice. Minoxidil is available over the counter and helps stimulate hair follicles and promote regrowth. Hair growth serums, like those containing biotin and caffeine, can also be effective. These serums nourish the scalp and strengthen hair follicles. Vitamins and supplements, such as those rich in biotin, zinc, and vitamin E, can support overall hair health. Brands like **Viviscal** and **Nutrafol** offer supplements specifically formulated for hair growth.

Making lifestyle changes can also support hair health. A balanced diet rich in vitamins and minerals is vital. Include plenty of leafy greens, nuts, seeds, and lean proteins in your meals. These foods provide the nutrients your hair needs to grow strong and healthy. Reducing stress through relaxation techniques like yoga, meditation, or even just taking a walk can make a big difference. Stress can wreak havoc on your hair, so finding ways to manage it is crucial. Avoiding harsh chemical treatments, like frequent dyeing or perming, can also help. These treatments can weaken your hair and contribute to thinning.

For more severe cases of hair loss, there are advanced treatments and options available. Platelet-rich plasma (PRP) therapy is one such treatment. It involves injecting your own platelet-rich plasma into your scalp to stimulate hair growth. Hair transplant surgery is another option. During this procedure, hair follicles are taken from one part of your scalp and transplanted to the thinning areas. Consulting a dermatologist or trichologist can provide you with personalized advice and treatment options. These professionals can help identify the underlying causes of your hair loss and recommend the best course of action.

Dealing with hair loss and thinning can be challenging, but understanding the causes and exploring various treatments can help you take control of the situation. Whether it's making lifestyle changes, using growth-promoting products, or seeking professional treatments, there are plenty of options to help you regain your hair's health and confidence.

7.7 Combating Heat Damage: Prevention And Repair

Let's talk about heat damage. Picture this: You've got your flat iron cranked up to the max, your blow-dryer blasting hot air like a dragon, and you're curling away like there's no tomorrow. While all that styling might make your hair look fabulous for the day, it's secretly plotting its revenge. High-temperature styling tools are the main culprits here. These bad boys can reach temperatures that literally fry your hair, making it dry, brittle, and prone to breakage. And if you're using these tools frequently without any protection, you're basically asking for trouble. Improper use, like not ensuring your hair is completely dry before applying heat, just adds fuel to the fire. It's like trying to iron wet clothes—never a good idea.

So, how do you shield your precious locks from turning into a crispy mess? Enter heat protectant sprays and serums. These products create a barrier between your hair and the heat, significantly reducing damage. A good one to try is the TRESemme Thermal Creations Heat Tamer Spray. It's lightweight, effective, and won't leave your hair feeling greasy. Leave-in conditioners with heat protection are also fantastic. They not only protect your hair but also keep it hydrated and smooth. Look for products that specifically mention heat protection on the label.

When it comes to heat styling, technique is everything. Start by using the lowest effective temperature setting on your tools. Just because your flat iron can go up to 450°F doesn't mean it should. Most hairstyles can be achieved at much lower temperatures, which are kinder to your hair. Limiting the frequency of heat styling is also crucial. Try to save those high-heat styles for special occasions and embrace your natural texture on other days. And always, always make sure your hair is completely dry before applying any heat. Wet hair and hot tools are a recipe for disaster. It's like trying to bake a cake in a microwave—sure, you can do it, but it won't end well.

If your hair has already suffered from heat damage, don't panic. There are plenty of treatments that can help bring it back to life. Start with deep conditioning treatments. These are your hair's best friend when it comes to hydration and repair. Look for masks that are rich in nourishing ingredients like shea butter or argan oil. Apply these treatments once a week to give your hair a moisture boost. Protein treatments can also work wonders. They help to rebuild the structure of your hair, making it stronger and more resilient. Products like Olaplex No. 3 Hair Perfector are designed to repair the bonds in your hair, restoring its strength and elasticity.

For an extra boost, consider using a leave-in conditioner or serum. These products provide ongoing hydration and protection, keeping your hair smooth and manageable throughout the day. Apply them to damp hair after washing and let them work their magic. Another great tip is to trim your hair regularly. Getting rid of those damaged ends can make your hair look and feel healthier instantly. It's like decluttering your room—sometimes, you need to let go of the old to make room for the new.

Heat damage might be a common issue, but it's not unbeatable. With the right products, techniques, and a little TLC, you can protect your hair from the perils of heat styling and keep it looking gorgeous. So go ahead and style away, but don't forget to treat your hair like the precious treasure it is.

7.8 Addressing Color Damage And Repairing Hair

Coloring your hair can be a fun way to switch up your look, but it often comes at a cost. Chemical damage is a major downside to dyes and bleaches. These chemicals are harsh and can break down the natural structure of your hair, making it more vulnerable to breakage. Bleaching, in particular, strips your hair of its natural pigment and weakens its overall strength. Moreover, color treatments can lead to a significant loss of moisture, leaving your hair feeling dry and straw-like. It's like turning a lush garden into a desert. The structural damage from these processes weakens the bonds within your hair, making it more prone to split ends and frizz. So, while that new shade might look amazing, it's essential to understand the toll it takes on your hair health.

Preventing color damage starts with making smarter choices during the coloring process. Opt for ammonia-free dyes whenever possible. Ammonia can be incredibly harsh, and ammonia-free options are gentler on your hair and scalp. Another good practice is to deep condition your hair before coloring it. This helps to fortify your strands, making them more resilient to the upcoming chemical assault. Also, try to avoid frequent color changes. Constantly switching shades means more chemical exposure, which can lead to cumulative damage. Stick to one color for a while and give your hair time to recover between treatments.

If your hair is already feeling the effects of color damage, don't worry—there are ways to repair it. Start with protein treatments. These products help to rebuild your hair's internal structure, making it stronger and more resilient. Hydrating masks are also essential. They restore the moisture that's been stripped away by coloring, leaving your hair soft and manageable. Products like Olaplex No. 3 Hair Perfector are fantastic for this. And, of course, sometimes you just need to cut your losses—literally. Trim the damaged ends to remove the worst of the damage and give your hair a fresh start.

Maintaining colored hair requires a little extra TLC. Use color-safe shampoos and conditioners to help preserve your shade and keep your hair healthy. These products are formulated to be gentle on your color while providing the necessary hydration and nutrients. Reducing heat styling is also crucial. Heat can further damage already weakened hair, so try to embrace air drying or use heat tools on a lower setting. Regular touch-ups are important to maintain color vibrancy, but try to limit them to every 6–8 weeks to avoid over-processing.

Coloring your hair can be a fun way to express yourself, but it's essential to take steps to protect it. From choosing gentler dyes to incorporating repairing treatments into your routine, there are plenty of ways to keep your hair looking vibrant and healthy. So go ahead and flaunt that new shade, but don't forget to give your hair the care it needs to stay fabulous.

CHAPTER 8: NATURAL HAIR CARE METHODS

Ever thought about raiding your kitchen for hair care products instead of your bathroom cabinet? It might sound a little odd, but trust me, natural oils can do wonders for your hair. Picture this: you're scrolling through Instagram, envying those glossy, luscious locks and wishing you could have the same. What if I told you that the secret to amazing hair might be sitting in your pantry right now? Forget fancy, overpriced products. Let's dive into the magic of natural oils and how they can transform your hair.

8.1 The Benefits Of Using Natural Oils For Hair

Alright, let's start with the superstar of natural hair care—coconut oil. This stuff is like a miracle in a jar. Coconut oil is packed with fatty acids that penetrate the hair shaft better than other oils, which means it's incredible for moisturizing. Say goodbye to dry, brittle hair and hello to silky, smooth strands. Plus, it's great for calming scalp irritation and fighting dandruff, thanks to its antifungal properties. Imagine giving your hair a hydrating boost while also tackling those pesky flakes. It's a win-win!

Next up, let's talk about castor oil. This thick, sticky oil might not look like much, but it's a heavyweight champion when it comes to strengthening your hair. It's rich in ricinoleic acid, which helps improve blood circulation to the scalp and promotes hair growth. If you're dreaming of longer, thicker locks, castor oil is your new best friend. And let's not forget tea tree oil. This little bottle of magic is fantastic for improving scalp health. With its antimicrobial properties, tea tree oil keeps your scalp clean and free from infections, making it the perfect solution for anyone dealing with itchiness or dandruff.

Now, let's get to know some other fabulous oils. Argan oil is often called "liquid gold," and for good reason. It's fantastic for adding shine and softness to your hair without making it greasy. If your hair is looking dull, a few drops of argan oil will bring it back to life. Jojoba oil is another gem. It closely mimics the natural oils produced by your scalp, which means it's excellent for balancing oil production. Whether your scalp is too oily or too dry, Jojoba oil can help bring it back into balance. And for those in need of deep conditioning, avocado oil is a must-try. It's rich in vitamins and nutrients that nourish your hair from the inside out, making it stronger and more resilient.

So, how do you use these oils to get the best results? Let's start with pre-shampoo treatments. Olive oil is fantastic for this. Warm a small amount and apply it to your hair, focusing on the ends. Leave it on for about 30 minutes before washing it out. This gives your hair a deep conditioning treatment and leaves it feeling soft and hydrated. For a leave-in conditioner, argan oil is your go-to. Just a few drops on damp hair will keep it moisturized and shiny all day long. And if you're looking for a relaxing scalp massage, almond oil is perfect. It's lightweight and easily absorbed, making it ideal for massaging into your scalp to improve blood circulation and promote hair growth.

8.2 Diy Oil Blend Recipes

Creating your own oil blends can be a fun and effective way to tailor treatments to your hair's specific needs. Here are a few simple recipes to get you started:
Hydrating Blend: Combine equal parts coconut oil and avocado oil. This blend is perfect for dry hair that needs a moisture boost. Apply it to your hair as a mask, leave it on for about 30 minutes,

and then wash it out.

Growth-Promoting Blend: Mix castor oil with a few drops of rosemary oil. This blend stimulates the scalp and promotes hair growth. Massage it into your scalp and let it sit for at least an hour before washing it out.

Anti-Frizz Blend: Combine argan oil and jojoba oil. This blend tames frizz and adds shine without weighing your hair down. Apply a small amount to damp hair and style as usual.

Using natural oils is a fantastic way to nourish, protect, and enhance your hair's health. These oils offer a range of benefits, from moisturizing and strengthening to improving scalp health. So next time you're thinking about how to give your hair some extra love, look no further than your kitchen. You might just find the perfect solution sitting right there.

8.3 Diy Natural Hair Treatments Using Kitchen Ingredients

Alright, let's get into the fun stuff—DIY hair treatments. Imagine whipping up a hair mask in your kitchen using ingredients you'd usually eat for breakfast. It's not just about feeling like a mad scientist; using natural kitchen ingredients for your hair has some serious perks. First off, you avoid harsh chemicals that can often be found in store-bought products. This means less irritation and more love for your scalp and hair. Plus, you can customize treatments to suit your specific needs. Have dry hair? There's a mask for that. Oily scalp? Got you covered. And let's not forget, these DIY treatments are super cost-effective. You're basically getting a spa treatment for the price of a banana and some honey.

Let's get into some recipes. If your hair is crying out for moisture, a honey and yogurt mask is your go-to. Honey is a natural humectant, which means it draws moisture into your hair. Yogurt, on the other hand, is packed with proteins and lactic acid that help to hydrate and strengthen your hair. To whip up this mask:

1. Mix two tablespoons of yogurt with one tablespoon of honey.
2. Apply it to your hair, focusing on the dry ends, and leave it on for about 20–30 minutes before rinsing. Your hair will feel soft and look shiny, like you've just had a professional treatment.

For those needing a bit of strength, the egg and olive oil treatment is a powerhouse. Eggs are protein-rich and help to rebuild and strengthen your hair shaft, while olive oil provides deep conditioning and shine.

1. Beat one egg and mix it with two tablespoons of olive oil. Apply the mixture evenly from roots to tips, ensuring every strand is coated.
2. Leave it on for about 15–20 minutes, and then rinse with cool water. Your hair will thank you for this protein boost and feel stronger and more resilient.

If you're dealing with an irritated or itchy scalp, the oatmeal and aloe vera remedy is a lifesaver. Oatmeal is soothing and helps to reduce inflammation, while aloe vera is hydrating and has antimicrobial properties.

1. Blend half a cup of oatmeal into a fine powder and mix it with two tablespoons of aloe vera gel.
2. Apply this paste to your scalp and let it sit for 20 minutes. Rinse thoroughly and enjoy a calm, soothed scalp.

When it comes to applying these treatments, there are a few tips to keep in mind. First, make sure to mix your ingredients to a smooth consistency. You don't want chunks of banana or clumps of oatmeal getting stuck in your hair. Use a blender or a whisk to get everything nicely combined. When applying, start from the roots and work your way to the tips, ensuring even coverage. Use your fingers or a brush to distribute the mask evenly. Leave the treatment on for the recommended time to allow the ingredients to work their magic before rinsing thoroughly.

Now, let's talk about potential allergens and sensitivities. It's super important to test any new treatment on a small patch of skin before slathering it all over your hair. This is called a patch test. Apply a small amount of the mixture to your inner wrist and wait 24 hours to see if there's any reaction. If your skin gets red or itchy, it's best to avoid that ingredient. Also, be aware of any known allergies. If you're allergic to nuts, steer clear of almond oil. If you have sensitive skin, consider diluting potent ingredients like tea tree oil with a carrier oil to minimize irritation.

Using DIY treatments is not only fun, but also incredibly beneficial for your hair. You can avoid harsh chemicals, customize treatments to your specific needs, and save money—all while treating your hair to some much-needed TLC. So, next time you're in the kitchen, take a look around and see what you can whip up for your hair. It might just become your new favorite self-care ritual.

8.4 Essential Oils For Hair Health: What To Use And How

Alright, let's talk about essential oils. These tiny bottles pack a punch when it comes to hair care. Essential oils are concentrated plant extracts with some serious powers.

Take tea tree oil, for example. This oil has antimicrobial properties that can keep your scalp clean and free from infections. If you've ever dealt with dandruff or an itchy scalp, tea tree oil can be a game-changer. It helps to unclog hair follicles and kill the bacteria or fungi that might be causing the problem.

Then there's peppermint oil, which is like a wake-up call for your scalp. It has stimulating effects that can increase blood circulation, promoting hair growth. The menthol in peppermint oil creates a tingling sensation, which feels lovely and helps invigorate your scalp.

And let's not forget about lavender oil. Known for its calming benefits, lavender oil can help reduce stress and improve overall scalp health. It also has antimicrobial properties, making it a double threat against scalp issues.

Choosing the right essential oil for your hair can be a bit like picking out candy from a shop—there are just so many good options! If you're looking to boost hair growth, rosemary oil is your go-to. It's known for improving cellular generation, which helps in thickening hair and promoting growth. For those with a sensitive scalp, chamomile oil is incredibly soothing. It helps calm irritation and can also add a beautiful shine to your hair. And if you're struggling with an oily scalp, lemon oil can help. It's great at balancing oil production and leaves your hair smelling fresh and clean.

Using essential oils isn't as simple as just pouring them onto your head, though. These oils are potent and need to be used correctly to avoid any issues. Always dilute essential oils with a carrier oil like coconut, almond, or jojoba oil. This helps to prevent irritation and ensures the oils are evenly distributed. A good rule of thumb is to mix about 3–5 drops of essential oil with a tablespoon of carrier oil. You can also add essential oils to your regular shampoo or conditioner. Just a few drops can enhance the benefits of your everyday products.

Scalp massages are another fantastic way to use essential oils. Not only do they feel incredible, but they also help improve blood circulation to your scalp, promoting hair growth. For a relaxing massage, mix lavender and chamomile oils with almond oil. Apply the blend to your scalp and massage gently for a few minutes. This nourishes your scalp and helps you unwind after a long day.

8.5 Diy Essential Oil Blend Recipes

Creating your own essential oil blends can be both fun and highly beneficial. Here are a few recipes to get you started:

Growth-Promoting Blend: Combine 5 drops of rosemary oil, 3 drops of peppermint oil, and 2 tablespoons of coconut oil. This blend stimulates the scalp and promotes hair growth. Massage it into your scalp and leave it on for at least an hour before washing it out.

Anti-Dandruff Blend: Mix 4 drops of tea tree oil, 3 drops of eucalyptus oil, and 2 tablespoons of olive oil. This blend helps to combat dandruff and keep your scalp healthy. Apply it to your scalp and let it sit for about 30 minutes before rinsing.

Relaxing Blend: Combine 5 drops of lavender oil, 3 drops of chamomile oil, and 2 tablespoons of almond oil. This blend is perfect for a soothing scalp massage that also promotes hair health. Massage it into your scalp and leave it on overnight for the best results.

Essential oils are a powerful addition to any hair care routine. They offer a range of benefits, from promoting growth to soothing the scalp and combating oiliness. By choosing the right oils and using them correctly, you can enhance your hair's health and appearance. So go ahead, experiment with these blends, and give your hair the love it deserves.

8.6 The Role Of Herbs And Botanicals In Hair Care

Ever thought about using herbs and botanicals for your hair? These natural wonders can make a huge difference in how your hair looks and feels. Take nettle, for example. It's not just a pesky weed; it's a powerhouse for hair health. Nettle is packed with vitamins and minerals that strengthen your hair from the roots, reducing breakage and promoting growth. Imagine your hair as a fortress and nettle as the bricks that make it strong and resilient.

Now, let's talk about hibiscus. This vibrant flower isn't just pretty to look at; it's a fantastic conditioner for your hair. Hibiscus helps to lock in moisture, making your hair softer and more manageable. Plus, it has natural antioxidants that protect your hair from environmental damage. Think of hibiscus as your hair's bodyguard, always on duty to keep it safe and smooth.

Chamomile is another gem in the botanical world. Known for its calming properties, chamomile can soothe an itchy, irritated scalp. It also adds a natural shine and highlights to your hair, making it look vibrant and healthy.

Rosemary is a superstar when it comes to stimulating hair growth. It improves blood circulation to the scalp, encouraging hair follicles to grow. If you're dreaming of long, luscious locks, rosemary could be your secret weapon.

Sage is another herb worth mentioning. It's excellent for enhancing hair color, especially if you have dark hair. Sage can deepen and enrich your natural color, giving it a glossy finish.

And then there's fenugreek. This herb is famous for reducing hair fall. Rich in proteins and nicotinic acid, fenugreek strengthens hair strands and promotes healthy growth. It's like giving your hair a protein shake, keeping it strong and full.

Incorporating these herbs into your hair care routine is easier than you might think. Herbal rinses are a great place to start. You can make a simple rinse with rosemary and nettle. Just steep the herbs in boiling water, let it cool, and pour it over your hair after shampooing. This rinse not only stimulates growth but also leaves your hair smelling amazing. Infused oils are another fantastic option. You can create an infused oil with hibiscus and lavender. Just add the herbs to a carrier oil like olive or coconut oil and let it sit for a few weeks. Use this infused oil as a hair mask or a scalp treatment to reap the benefits. And for a powerful hair mask, mix fenugreek seeds with aloe vera gel. This mask will nourish your scalp and reduce hair fall, leaving your hair looking and feeling its best.

8.7 Diy Herbal Hair Care Recipes

Creating your own herbal treatments at home are a fun and effective way to give your hair some extra love. Here are a few recipes to get you started:

Strengthening Rinse: Combine a handful of nettle and rosemary leaves in a pot of boiling water. Let it steep for about 30 minutes, then strain the liquid. After shampooing, pour this infusion over your hair and let it sit for a few minutes before rinsing with cool water.

Conditioning Mask: Blend hibiscus petals with coconut milk until you get a smooth paste. Apply this mask to your hair, focusing on the ends. Leave it on for 20–30 minutes, then rinse thoroughly. This mask will leave your hair feeling soft and deeply conditioned.

Scalp Soothing Treatment: Mix chamomile tea with aloe vera gel. Apply this mixture to your scalp and massage gently. Let it sit for about 15–20 minutes before rinsing. This treatment will calm any irritation and leave your scalp feeling refreshed.

Herbs and botanicals are like nature's gift to your hair. They offer a range of benefits, from strengthening and conditioning to improving scalp health. Plus, they're easy to incorporate into your routine with simple, homemade treatments. So next time you're thinking about how to pamper your hair, look no further than your garden or kitchen. You might just find the perfect solution right there.

8.8 Creating Your Own Natural Hair Care Products

Imagine opening your bathroom cabinet and being greeted not by a slew of plastic bottles filled with unpronounceable ingredients, but by a few simple, homemade hair care products tailored just for you. Making your own hair care products allows you to customize formulations to meet your specific needs. No more guessing whether that store-bought shampoo will work for your oily scalp or if that conditioner will tame your frizz. You can whip up exactly what your hair craves, avoiding synthetic chemicals and preservatives that can often do more harm than good. Plus, it's a cost-effective and environmentally friendly way to take care of your hair. Ready to become a hair care alchemist? Let's get started.

First up, let's talk about making your own shampoo. You'll need Castile soap, coconut milk, and essential oils. Castile soap is a natural, vegetable-based soap that's gentle yet effective at cleansing. Coconut milk adds moisture and nutrients, while essential oils like lavender or peppermint can provide additional benefits like soothing the scalp or promoting hair growth. To make your shampoo, mix one cup of Castile soap with one cup of coconut milk. Add 20–30 drops of your favorite essential oils. Pour the mixture into a bottle and shake well before each use. This shampoo not only cleanses your hair but also leaves it feeling soft and nourished.

Now, let's move on to a DIY conditioner. You'll need shea butter, avocado oil, and aloe vera. Shea butter is fantastic for deep conditioning, avocado oil is rich in nutrients, and aloe vera provides hydration and soothing properties. To make your conditioner, melt half a cup of shea butter in a double boiler. Once melted, remove from heat and add two tablespoons of avocado oil and half a cup of aloe vera gel. Whisk until well combined and let it cool. Apply this conditioner to your hair after shampooing, focusing on the ends. Leave it on for a few minutes before rinsing thoroughly. Your hair will feel incredibly soft and manageable.

For a leave-in treatment, aloe vera gel, glycerin, and lavender oil are your best friends. Aloe vera gel hydrates and soothes, glycerin helps to retain moisture, and lavender oil adds a calming scent while promoting hair health. Mix half a cup of aloe vera gel with two tablespoons of glycerin and 10 drops of lavender oil. Pour the mixture into a spray bottle and shake well. Spray this leave-in treatment on damp hair, focusing on the mid-lengths and ends. It will keep your hair moisturized and smelling divine throughout the day.

Formulating effective hair care products isn't just about mixing ingredients. You need to ensure they are safe and effective. Balancing pH levels in your homemade shampoo is crucial. Hair has a natural pH of around 4.5 to 5.5, so your shampoo should be slightly acidic to match this. You can test the pH level using pH strips and adjust it by adding a few drops of apple cider vinegar if needed. Preserving your natural products is also important. Essential oils add fragrance and benefits and have antimicrobial properties that help preserve the product. When making conditioners, ensure proper emulsification by blending ingredients thoroughly. This enables the oils and water-based ingredients to mix well, giving you a smooth and effective product.

Storing your homemade products properly ensures they stay fresh and effective. Use dark glass bottles to preserve the ingredients and protect them from light. Label each product with the ingredients and the date it was made, so you know what's in it and when to use it by. Before applying any new product to your whole head, test it on a small area to ensure you don't have an allergic reaction. This simple step can save you from potential irritation and disappointment.

Creating your own natural hair care products is not only fun, but also incredibly rewarding. You get to tailor each product to your specific needs, avoid harmful chemicals, and save money, all while being kind to the environment. So, roll up your sleeves and start experimenting with these recipes. Your hair will thank you.

8.9 Going Green: Sustainable And Eco-Friendly Hair Care Practices

Let's talk about something super important—sustainability in hair care. You might be thinking, "Why should I care about sustainability when it comes to my hair?" Well, adopting eco-friendly practices is not only great for the planet but also beneficial for your hair. For starters, reducing plastic waste from hair care products is a big win. Imagine all those empty shampoo bottles piling up in landfills. By switching to more sustainable options, you're doing your bit to reduce that plastic mountain. Plus, many eco-friendly products minimize exposure to harmful chemicals, which means your hair gets all the benefits without the nasty side effects. And let's not forget about supporting ethical and sustainable brands. By choosing these products, you're endorsing companies that are committed to protecting the environment and treating their workers fairly. It's a win-win for everyone involved.

So, what are some sustainable hair care products you can use? Solid shampoo bars are a fantastic option. They come with minimal packaging, last longer than liquid shampoos, and are just as effective at keeping your hair clean and fresh. Brands like Ethique and Lush offer a range of shampoo bars that cater to different hair types. Another great option is biodegradable hair ties. These are made from natural materials that break down faster than traditional plastic or rubber hair ties. Look for brands like Kooshoo, which makes biodegradable hair ties in various colors. And if you're into reducing waste further, check out refillable product options. Many companies now offer refill stations or mail-in refills for their products. It's a great way to keep using your favorite products without constantly buying new bottles.

Reducing waste in your daily hair care routine doesn't have to be complicated. Start by using reusable tools like bamboo brushes. Bamboo is a sustainable material that's gentle on your hair and the environment. Plus, bamboo brushes look super chic on your vanity. Another tip is to make DIY hair products in small batches. This way, you only make what you need, reducing waste and ensuring your products are always fresh. And when it comes to finished products, don't just throw away the containers. Recycling and upcycling product containers can be a fun and creative way to reduce waste. Turn an old shampoo bottle into a cute planter for your succulents, or use it to store craft supplies. The possibilities are endless.

Being mindful of your choices can have a significant impact. When shopping for hair care products, look for those with eco-friendly packaging. Brands that use recyclable or biodegradable materials for their packaging are making a conscious effort to reduce waste. Supporting brands with ethical sourcing practices is another way to make a difference. These companies ensure that the ingredients they use are sustainability sourced and that the workers involved in production are treated fairly. Participating in recycling programs for hair care products is also a great way to contribute. Some brands, like Lush, offer incentives for returning empty containers, which they then recycle or re-purpose.

Making sustainable choices isn't just about what's good for the environment; it's also about what's good for you. Eco-friendly hair care products often use natural ingredients that are gentler on your hair and scalp. By reducing your exposure to harmful chemicals, you're promoting healthier hair in the long run. Plus, supporting ethical brands means you're contributing to a fairer, more sustainable world. It's a small change that can make a big difference. So, next time you're shopping for hair care products, think about how your choices can impact the planet and your hair. You've got the power to make a positive change, one bottle at a time.

CHAPTER 9: INSPIRING CONFIDENCE AND CREATIVITY

Have you ever felt like your hair is an extension of who you are? Like it's your own personal billboard, announcing your mood, your style, and even your values? Trust me, you're not alone. Hair is more than just strands of protein—it's a powerful tool for self-expression. Think about it: when you're rocking a killer hairstyle, don't you just feel more confident? Like you could take on the world? That's because your hair is a reflection of your personality, mood, and, yes, even your lifestyle.

9.1 Finding Your Personal Style: Hair As A Form Of Self-Expression

Your hair can say so much about you. It can reflect your personality, whether you're the life of the party or the quiet thinker. It can mirror your mood. Have you ever noticed how you tend to wear it up when you're feeling a bit meh, or down when you're in a relaxed mood? Your hairstyle can also align with your values and lifestyle. Maybe you're all about sustainability, so you choose eco-friendly hair products. Or perhaps you're super busy, so you opt for low-maintenance styles that still look fab. Whatever the case, your hair is a canvas, and you're the artist.

So, how do you discover your personal style? Start with creating a mood board. Grab some magazines, or better yet, hop on Pinterest and start pinning looks that catch your eye. This visual collection will help you see patterns and preferences you might not have noticed before. Next, it's time to experiment. Try different styles and colors. Don't be afraid to step out of your comfort zone. Maybe you've always wanted to try a bold color or rock some edgy bangs. Now's your chance! Remember to consider your face shape and hair type when exploring new styles. What looks good on a heart-shaped face might not have the same effect on a round one, so tailor your choices to what enhances your natural features.

Inspiration is everywhere. Look to your cultural heritage for traditional styles that can be modernized. Draw inspiration from your favorite celebrities and influencers. They often set trends that trickle down to the rest of us, so why not take a page out of their book? Artistic and fashion trends can also influence your hair choices. Just like fashion, hair trends evolve, and incorporating these elements can keep your look fresh and current.

Embrace change and be open to experimentation. Temporary changes like wigs and extensions are great for trying out a new look without the commitment. Seasonal styles can keep things exciting. Maybe rock beachy waves in the summer and sleek, straight hair in the winter. Don't be afraid to seek feedback from friends and family. Sometimes an outside perspective can help you see what really works for you.

9.2 Interactive Element: Create Your Hair Mood Board

Grab a stack of old magazines, or open your Pinterest app. Start collecting images of hairstyles, colors, and vibes that you're drawn to. Arrange them in a collage. This mood board will be your go-to source of inspiration when you're ready to switch up your style. Reflect on why you chose each image. Is it the color? The cut? The texture? Understanding your preferences will help you make more confident styling choices.

So, what's your hair saying about you? Is it reflecting the confident, creative person you are, or is it time for a refresh? Remember, your hair is a powerful tool for self-expression. Use it to show the world who you are and who you're becoming.

9.3 Hair Care And Styling For Different Occasions

Ever wondered why your hair looks amazing for a night out but falls flat for a job interview? It's all about occasion-specific hairstyles. Just like you wouldn't wear a ball gown to the grocery store, your hair needs to match the vibe of the event you're attending. Different settings call for different styles, and getting it right can boost your confidence and make you feel like you've nailed the occasion.

Professional settings demand polished, professional looks. Think sleek low buns and ponytails that keep your hair out of your face while looking super chic. Minimalist braids and twists also work wonders here. They're neat and tidy and show you mean business. Subtle accessories like hairpins and clips can add a touch of personality without going overboard. The key is to keep it simple yet sophisticated so you look professional without sacrificing style. Whether it's a job interview or a big presentation, these styles will have you looking sharp and ready to impress.

Casual outings and everyday wear give you more room to play around. Messy buns and top knots are lifesavers on days when you want to look cute but can't be bothered with a complicated style. They're quick, easy, and effortlessly stylish. Low-maintenance braids and twists are perfect for adding a bit of flair without much effort. Simple half-up, half-down styles are versatile and can transition from a casual coffee date to a day at the mall. These styles keep you looking fresh and put together without demanding too much time or effort.

Special occasions like weddings, parties, and formal events call for a bit more glam. Romantic curls and waves are always a hit. They add volume and movement, making you feel like a Hollywood starlet. Intricate updos and chignons bring an air of elegance. They can seem daunting, but with a bit of practice, you can create stunning styles that turn heads. Adding accessories like flowers, headbands, or jewels can elevate your look even further. These little touches can make your hairstyle look more polished and event-appropriate.

Adding accessories can transform a simple hairstyle into something special. Flowers can add a romantic touch to curls or braids. Headbands can give your look a vintage vibe, while jewels can make you feel like a princess. Don't be afraid to experiment with different accessories to see what works best for you. They can add that final touch that takes your hairstyle from everyday to extraordinary.

So, whether you're heading to a job interview, a casual outing, or a formal event, having a few go-to hairstyles can make all the difference. Matching your hair to the occasion completes your look and boosts your confidence. You'll walk in feeling prepared and looking fabulous, no matter where you're headed.

9.4 Building Confidence In Your Hair Styling Abilities

Ever felt a wave of panic trying a new hairstyle, convinced you'll end up looking like a walking disaster? You're not alone. Confidence in hairstyling can totally transform how you feel about yourself. It's all about overcoming that fear of messing up and embracing the process. Mistakes? They're just part of the learning curve. Seriously, no one gets it right the first time. And guess what? That's perfectly okay. Every little victory, like nailing a simple braid or mastering a tricky bun, is worth celebrating. These small successes build up your confidence bit by bit.

To start building your hairstyling confidence, practice is key. Begin with basic styles. Get comfy with a simple ponytail or a three-strand braid. Once you've got those down, gradually step up your game. Try more advanced techniques like fishtail braids or intricate updos. The more you practice, the more natural it will feel. And don't shy away from seeking feedback. Ask friends or family for their honest opinions. Constructive feedback can be a goldmine for improvement. Remember, everyone started as a beginner.

Staying motivated can sometimes be a challenge, but there are ways to keep the excitement alive. Follow inspiring hair accounts on social media. Seeing others' creativity can spark your own. Set personal hairstyling goals, whether it's mastering a new technique each month or experimenting with different accessories. Joining online communities or forums can also provide a sense of camaraderie. You're not just styling your hair alone; you're part of a bigger community that shares your passion and supports your growth.

And hey, don't forget to be your own cheerleader. Sometimes you need a little boost to keep going. Remember these affirmations: "Your hair is your crown; wear it with pride." Every time you try a new style, remind yourself, "Every great style starts with a single step." And most importantly, "Believe in your skills and the beauty you create." These words can be your mantra when you're feeling unsure. They're a reminder that you're capable and that your efforts are worth it.

Building confidence in your hairstyling abilities is a journey filled with ups and downs. But with each attempt, you get better, and with each success, your confidence grows. So, grab your brushes, your hair ties, and your bobby pins because you're ready to create something amazing.

9.5 Success Stories: Real-Life Testimonials And Inspirations

Imagine hearing about someone who faced the same hair struggles you do and came out the other side with fabulous, healthy hair. There's something incredibly inspiring about real-life success stories. They remind us that we're not alone in our hair challenges and that with a bit of perseverance, we can achieve our hair goals. Relatable experiences, overcoming obstacles, and celebrating diverse hair journeys can motivate you like nothing else. Let's dive into some fantastic stories from individuals who have transformed their hair care routines and styling skills.

One story that stands out is from a friend who decided to transition to natural hair. She battled years of damage from chemical relaxers and heat styling. The journey wasn't easy—there were awkward lengths, bad hair days, and many moments of doubt. But she stuck with it, embracing her natural curls and learning how to care for them properly. Today, her hair is healthy, bouncy, and full of life. She feels more like herself than ever before and loves the confidence that comes with embracing her natural texture.

Then there's the tale of someone who mastered complex styles through sheer determination. A young woman I know was always fascinated by intricate braids and updos but felt intimidated by their complexity. She started small, practicing basic braids until she could do them in her sleep. Gradually, she moved on to more complicated styles, like fishtail braids and crown braids. Now, she can whip up an intricate updo in no time, and her friends often ask her to style their hair for special occasions. Her journey shows that practice and patience can lead to mastering even the most challenging styles.

Achieving hair health goals is another common theme in these success stories. One individual struggled with dry, brittle hair for years. She decided to overhaul her hair care routine, focusing on hydration and nourishment. She incorporated deep conditioning treatments, avoided heat styling, and used natural oils to keep her hair moisturized. Over time, her hair transformed from brittle and lifeless to soft and shiny. She couldn't believe the difference and now shares her tips with anyone who will listen.

These stories come from people with a variety of hair types and styles. Curly and coily hair, for instance, often requires a different approach than straight or wavy hair. One curly-haired friend shared how she finally found a routine that works for her after years of using products that left her hair frizzy and undefined. She discovered the magic of leave-in conditioners and styling gels and learned to embrace her curls. Her hair is now a source of pride, and she loves experimenting with different curly styles.

On the other end of the spectrum, a friend with straight hair struggled with volume and flatness. She learned techniques to add body and bounce, like using volumizing products and mastering the art of the blowout. Her hair now has the volume she always dreamed of, and she feels confident in any setting. Another friend with wavy hair found that scrunching her hair with a sea salt spray gave her the beachy waves she always wanted without the need for a curling iron.

Short hair poses its own set of challenges and opportunities. One individual decided to chop off her long locks and go for a pixie cut. The change was drastic, but she embraced it fully. She learned new styling techniques and found that short hair can be just as versatile as long hair. She now switches up her look with ease, using products to add texture and definition. Her confidence soars and she loves the edgy vibe her short hair gives her.

These testimonials are just a few examples of how diverse hair journeys can be. From transitioning to natural hair to mastering complex styles, each story is unique and inspiring. I encourage you to share your own experiences and inspire others. Whether it's on social media, in future editions of this book, or in online forums, your story can motivate someone else to take control of their hair health and styling skills. Celebrate your victories, big or small, and become part of a community that supports and uplifts each other.

9.6 Social Media Influencers To Follow For Hair Inspiration

Ever find yourself lost in an Instagram scroll, mesmerized by flawless hair transformations, and wondering how the heck they do it? Social media influencers have turned platforms like Instagram, TikTok, and YouTube into treasure troves of hair inspiration. They showcase diverse styles and techniques, giving you endless ideas to experiment with. Whether it's a new braid, a sassy updo, or even a daring color change, influencers are at the forefront of hair trends. They also offer product recommendations and reviews, helping you navigate the overwhelming world of hair care products. Trust me, their tutorials and how-to guides can turn even the most hair-challenged among us into styling pros.

If you've got curly or coily hair, you need to check out influencers who specialize in natural textures. **Nià**, the founder of **The Curl Bar London**, is a must-follow. She's all about embracing natural curls and offers tons of tutorials on how to care for and style curly hair. **Negin Mirsalehi**, founder of **Gisou**, is a fantastic source of inspiration for straight and wavy hair. Her sleek, glossy waves are the stuff of hair dreams. And if you're into DIY hair care, **Cynthia Dhimdis** is your go-to. She's known for her effortless, trending hairstyles and practical advice for maintaining healthy hair at home.

What makes these influencers worth following? It's not just their amazing hair. It's their innovative styling techniques, engaging and educational content, and positive, inclusive messaging. Nià's tutorials are not only super helpful but also incredibly empowering. She encourages followers to love their natural hair and provides practical tips to make it look its best. Negin's content is a mix of glamorous hair inspiration and down-to-earth advice. She shares everything from her favorite products to her go-to styling hacks. Cynthia's engaging tutorials make even the most complicated styles seem achievable. She's all about making hair care accessible and fun.

Engaging with influencers can take your hair game to the next level. Don't be shy about asking questions or seeking advice. Most influencers are more than happy to help and often respond to comments and DMs. Participating in live tutorials and Q&A sessions can provide real-time feedback and tips. It's like having a personal hair coach! Supporting influencers by liking, sharing, and commenting boosts their visibility and keeps you in the loop with the latest trends and techniques.

9.7 Interactive Element: Follow And Engage With Influencers

Grab your phone and follow a few hair influencers that resonate with you. Start with **Nià**, **Negin MirsalehI**, and **Cynthia Dhimdis**. Spend some time exploring their content. Leave thoughtful comments, ask questions, and participate in their live sessions. Take note of any tips or products they recommend. Try incorporating some of their advice into your hair routine and see how it works for you.

In a world where hair care can feel overwhelming, influencers simplify the process and make it enjoyable. They bring fresh ideas, practical tips, and a sense of community to your hair journey. So hit that follow button, and let these hair guru's guide you to your best hair days.

9.8 The Future Of Hair Care: Trends And Innovations

Ever wondered what the future holds for hair care? Spoiler alert: it's pretty exciting. The world of hair care is evolving, and there are some seriously cool trends and innovations on the horizon. First off, sustainable and eco-friendly products are taking center stage. Gone are the days when you had to choose between great hair and saving the planet. Today, more brands are focusing on eco-friendly packaging, cruelty-free formulas, and natural ingredients. This shift not only benefits the environment but also your hair, reducing exposure to harsh chemicals and promoting overall health.

Next up, personalized hair care solutions are revolutionizing the way we approach hair health. Imagine having a product line tailored specifically to your hair type, texture, and even your scalp condition. Companies are now using advanced technology to create bespoke hair care regimens. Think customized shampoos, conditioners, and treatments that address your unique needs. It's like having a personal stylist in a bottle. This trend is all about making hair care more effective and personalized, taking the guesswork out of choosing the right products.

Technological advancements in hair tools are also making waves. From smart hair brushes that analyze your hair health to high-tech straighteners that adjust the temperature based on your hair type, the future of hair tools is all about precision and care. These innovations aim to minimize damage while maximizing results, giving you salon-quality hair at home. It's like having a team of hair experts in your bathroom, ensuring you get the best possible outcome every time you style your hair.

Let's discuss some innovative hair care techniques that are gaining popularity. **Scalp microneedling** is one of those cutting-edge methods that are making a buzz. This technique involves tiny needles creating micro-injuries on the scalp, stimulating hair growth, and improving overall scalp health. It might sound a bit intense, but many swear by its effectiveness. **Cryotherapy** is another cool (literally) treatment that's catching on. This involves using freezing temperatures to boost hair health, reduce frizz, and increase shine. Advanced hair repair treatments using ingredients like keratin and biotin are also becoming more sophisticated, offering a deeper, more effective repair for damaged hair.

Industry experts have plenty to say about these trends. Leading hair care professionals predict that the focus on sustainability and personalization will only grow stronger. Innovations in hair care science, such as the development of new ingredients and technologies, are set to transform how we think about hair health. There's also a significant shift towards inclusivity and diversity in the industry. Brands are recognizing the importance of catering to all hair types and textures, ensuring that everyone can find products and treatments that work for them.

Staying informed about these trends and innovations is easier than you might think. Following reputable hair care blogs and publications is a great way to keep your finger on the pulse. Websites like **NaturallyCurly** and **Allure** often feature the latest in hair care news and product reviews. Attending hair care and beauty events in person or virtually can also provide valuable insights and inspiration. These events often feature industry experts, product launches, and live demonstrations. Joining online hair care communities, like Reddit's **HaircareScience** or various Facebook groups, can also be incredibly helpful. These platforms allow you to connect with fellow hair enthusiasts, share tips, and stay updated on the latest trends.

So, whether you're passionate about sustainability, excited about personalized products, or curious about the latest technology, the future of hair care has something for everyone. It's an exciting time to be a hair enthusiast, with endless possibilities for healthier, more beautiful hair. By staying informed and open to new ideas, you can take full advantage of these innovations and keep your hair looking and feeling its best.

As we wrap up this chapter, remember that the future of hair care is bright and full of possibilities. From sustainable products to high-tech tools, there's a world of innovation waiting to be explored. Stay curious, stay informed, and most importantly, have fun with your hair. In the next chapter, we'll dive into some practical tips and tricks to make your hair care routine even more effective.

CONCLUSION

Hey there, hair care hero! Can you believe we've reached the end of our hair journey together? It's been quite the ride, hasn't it? From understanding your hair's anatomy to mastering the art of various styles, we've covered a lot of ground. But before you close this book and go rock your fabulous hair, let's take a moment to wrap things up.

First off, let's recap the main points we've tackled. We started by diving into the basics of hair structure and growth. Remember the medulla, cortex, and cuticle? Like a tiny tree, your hair has layers that need love and care. We then identified your hair type —straight, wavy, curly, or coily—and how that influences your hair care routine. Scalp health was another biggie, with tips on maintaining a healthy scalp to ensure your hair grows strong and shiny. And who could forget the fun we had with different hair porosity levels? Low, medium, high—each has its quirks and needs.

We didn't stop there. We ventured into building a healthy hair care routine, focusing on daily, weekly, and monthly habits that keep your hair in tip-top shape. We covered everything from daily moisturizing sprays to weekly deep conditioning sessions. And we even discussed the importance of protecting your hair while you sleep. Silk pillowcases, anyone?

Then, we got into the nitty-gritty of hair-washing techniques and tips. How often should you wash your hair? What shampoo and conditioner should you use? We answered these burning questions and more. And let's not forget the styling techniques we explored. From basic ponytails to intricate braids and elegant chignons, you're now equipped to handle any hair situation that comes your way.

And hey, remember those protective styles and maintenance tips? Box braids, twists, and even wigs—they're all fantastic ways to give your hair a break while still looking fabulous. We also tackled common hair problems like frizz, breakage, and split ends, offering solutions and remedies to keep your hair healthy and happy.

Now, let's talk about the key takeaways. First and foremost, understanding your hair is the foundation of effective hair care. Knowledge is power, and now you have the tools to make informed decisions about your hair. Consistency is crucial. Small, regular actions lead to long-term benefits. Whether it's daily moisturizing or weekly deep conditioning, sticking to a routine makes all the difference. And please remember the importance of a balanced diet. Healthy hair starts from within, so nourish your body to nourish your hair.

So, what's next? Well, it's time to put all this knowledge into action. Start by evaluating your current hair care routine. What's working? What's not? Make adjustments based on what you've learned. Experiment with new styles and techniques. Don't be afraid to try something new. Whether it's a bold new color or a fancy updo, have fun with your hair. And most importantly, share your journey. Inspire others by sharing your tips, tricks, and successes. You never know who might benefit from your experience.

Before we part ways, I want to leave you with a final thought. Your hair is more than just strands of protein. It's a reflection of who you are, your personality, and your creativity. Embrace it, love it, and take pride in it. Every day is a new opportunity to express yourself through your hair. So go ahead, hold your head high, and let your hair tell your story.

Thank you for joining me on this journey. I hope this book has been as fun and informative for you as it was for me to write. Now, go out there and rock those gorgeous locks! You've got this.

Sophia Forbes

REFERENCES

- *Physiology, Hair - StatPearls - NCBI Bookshelf* https://www.ncbi.nlm.nih.gov/books/NBK499948/#:~:text=This%20cycle%20can%20be%20divided,into%20proanagen%20and%20metanagen%20phases.
- *Hormonal Effects on Hair Follicles - PMC* https://www.ncbi.nlm.nih.gov/pmc/articles/PMC7432488/
- *Curly Hair Types Chart: How to Find Your Curl Pattern | Allure* https://www.allure.com/gallery/curl-hair-type-guide#:~:text=Identifying%20your%20curl%20shape%20and,wave%2C%20curl%2C%20or%20coil.
- *Scalp Condition Impacts Hair Growth and Retention via ...* https://www.ncbi.nlm.nih.gov/pmc/articles/PMC6369642/
- *Hair Care Routine Steps for Healthy Hair* https://us.gisou.com/blogs/blog/hair-care-routine-steps
- *Goodbye, Dry Hair: Here's How to Deep Condition at Home ...* https://www.healthline.com/health/beauty-skin-care/how-to-deep-condition-hair
- *How Often Should You Actually Cut Your Hair?* https://www.healthline.com/health/beauty-skin-care/how-often-should-you-cut-your-hair
- *Satin vs. Silk Pillowcases for Hair: What's the Difference?* https://www.byrdie.com/satin-pillowcase-for-hair-5189103
- *How Often Should You Wash Your Hair?* https://www.healthline.com/health/beauty-skin-care/how-

- often-should-you-wash-your-hair#:~:text=Most%20people%20don't%20need,feels%20unclean%20to%20the%20touch.
- *The 15 Best Shampoos for Curly Hair, Tested & Reviewed* https://www.instyle.com/best-shampoos-for-curly-hair-8652537
- *How to Co-Wash Hair and Why It Works, According to Experts* https://www.realsimple.com/beauty-fashion/hair/hair-care/co-wash-natural-hair
- *8 Common Hair Washing Mistakes and How to Correct Them* https://www.byrdie.com/mistakes-people-make-when-shampooing-their-hair-345624
- *What Type of Hairbrush is Best for Your Hair? - Healthline* https://www.healthline.com/health/hair-brush-types#:~:text=Tiny%20boar%20bristle%20brush&text=Every%20type%20of%20hair%20can,%2C%20thinning%2C%20or%20aging%20hair.
- *31 Easy Ponytail Hairstyles to Try At Home* https://www.ipsy.com/blog/easy-ponytail-hairstyles
- *How to Braid Hair: 10 Techniques (With Videos)* https://www.wikihow.com/Braid-Hair
- *4 Ways to Get Curls without Heat and the Benefits of Using ...* https://www.shopnhe.com/blogs/press-media/ways-to-get-curls-without-heat-and-the-benefits-of-using-heatless-curl-methods
- *A Complete Guide to French Braiding Hair* https://www.wikihow.com/French-Braid
- *How to Give Yourself a Salon-Worthy Blowout at Home* https://www.allure.com/story/at-home-blowout
- *20 Ways to Get Creative with Your Hair Accessories* https://www.herstyler.com/20-ways-to-get-creative-with-hair-ornamentation/
- *Heat Style Your Hair with Bea Carmichael* https://www.aveda.ca/how-to-heat-style-with-bea-carmichael

- *Protective Hairstyles Benefits: Here's What You ... - Garnier* https://www.garnierusa.com/tips-how-tos/what-are-protective-hairstyles-and-why-are-they-good-for-you
- *How to do box braids at home: a step-by-step guide* https://www.luxyhair.com/blogs/hair-blog/how-to-do-box-braids?srsltid=AfmBOorQS3DZ3kGfVlH0kh7joXzuWF-SCLmxW2Gi7Z7uLfPN2tW1W_ig
- *The Best Products for Rope Twists on Natural Hair* https://www.beautycon.com/article/the-best-products-for-rope-twists-on-natural-hair
- *How to Choose the Right Wig: A Comprehensive Guide* https://www.bravadas.com/about/blog/how-to-choose-the-right-wig-a-comprehensive-guide.html
- *6 Surprising Causes of Frizzy Hair – and 8 Ways to Combat It* https://www.healthline.com/health/beauty-skin-care/what-causes-frizzy-hair
- *How to Stop Hair Breakage: Causes, Signs & Prevention* https://www.livingproof.com/hair-101/hair-breakage.html
- *How to Fix Split Ends, According to Hair Stylists* https://www.byrdie.com/diy-split-end-remedies-4795825
- *9 Best Dry Scalp Treatments of 2024, According to ...* https://www.cosmopolitan.com/style-beauty/beauty/g30896457/dry-scalp-treatment-products/
- *Coconut Oil for Hair Growth: Research, Efficacy, and More* https://www.healthline.com/health/beauty-skin-care/coconut-oil-for-hair-growth
- *15 Best DIY Hair Masks of 2024* https://www.goodhousekeeping.com/beauty/hair/g29627145/diy-hair-masks/
- *9 Essential Oils for Hair Growth & Health* https://www.healthline.com/health/essential-oils-for-hair-growth
- *19 Herbal Remedies for Hair Growth* https://

www.healthline.com/health/herbs-for-hair-growth
- *Using Hairstyles to Express Your Inner Self* https://discover.hubpages.com/style/Using-Hairstyles-to-Express-Your-Inner-Self
- *30 Formal Hairstyles for Special Occasion in 2024* https://therighthairstyles.com/hairstyles-for-special-occasions/
- *Understanding the Powerful Connection Between Hair and ...* https://www.spornette.com/powerful-connection-between-hair-and-confidence/
- *Top 50 Hair Influencers in 2024* https://influencers.feedspot.com/hair_care_instagram_influencers/
- French Braid vs Dutch braid (With Step-By-Step Picture Guide) https://www.hairqueenie.com/blogs/news/french-braid-vs-dutch-braid
- Everyday Hair inspiration https://www.everydayhairinspiration.com/2019/08/31/3-strand-braid/#google_vignette
- How To Do An Easy Fishtail Braid.https://www.musely.com/tips/How-To-Do-An-Easy-Fishtail-Braid/10679707?u=MTM5NjkxOTYwMHwyfHB0fDE4NTg0Mjd8MTA2Nzk3MDd8MjAxNDA0MjktMDcwMA&epik=dj0yJnU9NjlHR3VTM2pDZzI2VFgxajNVMWVGc3B1dGVEdUNvdTYmcD0wJm49aXVpbndlLXNfQXV4eVItWVBBJZjI5QSZ0PUFBQUFBR2JmSm5v
- Three Strand Waterfall Braids Tutorial https://lynetteemakeup.blogspot.com/2016/03/three-strand-waterfall-braids-tutorial.html
- Hair type and know how to style yours https://therighthairstyles.com/hair-types/

Printed in Dunstable, United Kingdom